The Tibetan Art of Healing

BY

Theodore Burang

WATKINS · LONDON

Publishers & Booksellers

First published text *Tibetische Heilkunde*
Printed in Switzerland 1957
© by Origo Verlag Zurich

First Impression 1974

Produced and distributed by
Watkins Publishing
45 Lower Belgrave Street
London SW1W 0LT
England
in association with Watkins Bookshop
21 Cecil Court
Charing Cross Road
London WC2N 4HB

Text designed and printed at
The Compton Press Ltd.
Compton Chamberlayne
Salisbury, Wiltshire

SBN 7224 0134 5

Contents

Translator's Preface

DURING the work of translating this book, I read extensively around the subject. The god of modern Western medical science and engineering technology does not appear to be living up to expectations. Awareness is growing of other factors which play a part in man's existence: the earth's ecology, emotional and spiritual aspects of his being, and subtle spheres, which are beginning to be accepted now that more refined instruments are being developed for their detection.

Due to his lack of awareness up to now, Western man has been rushing in where angels fear to tread, with the best intentions, of course. And not only at home. His ignorance and fear of death mean that he values short-term cures most, and is in a desperate hurry to do as much as he can, both to stave off the unknown in the present and to fulfil his life in the best way he knows, before the inevitable day arrives.

Almost any system can be applied either constructively or destructively, and the Tibetan medical system is no exception. Even the Chinese, who seem to be effectively integrating the ancient and modern, are gradually exterminating the spiritual element of Tibetan life. It seems that all-seeing, impartial observers are needed to sort out what is real and beneficial to mankind from what is not.

However, since such people are sadly lacking, let us at least retain an open mind to the possibility that there might be some realistic basis for Tibetan 'superstitions'.

SUSAN MACINTOSH

Author's Preface

THE MEDICINE indigenous to Tibet is highly respected throughout central Asia and has a remarkable record of success in healing. Its philosophy and curative methods transport us into a strange web of macrocosmic and microcosmic interrelations. In contrast to the standpoint of Western research, it acquaints us with unusual spiritual foundations – derived in part from ancient Indian philosophy – and often displays a masterful observation of nature. My intensive studies of the Tibetan language which, because it is so extraordinarily difficult, spanned many years, enabled me to study various principal works of the extensive medical literature of Tibet. Interest in this hitherto little-known field has grown over the years, and its practical significance has become increasingly recognised. This is due to the publication of contributions about this traditional school of Asian medicine in many journals all over the world.

It has not been easy to give a general outline of the whole picture of Tibetan medicine in a small book. Thus apart from two sections written in greater depth, I have only been able to give as much detail as seems necessary for the reader's understanding of the subject as a whole.

THEODORE BURANG

The Cosmic Humours

TIBETAN medicine enjoys a very high reputation, not only in Tibet itself, but also amongst many millions throughout central Asia. Considering its indisputable success in curing disease, it is hard to believe that the West, with its proverbial pragmatism and thirst for knowledge, has hesitated for so long to come to grips with a system of healing of such renown. This is partly due to the fact that eminent healers tend not to proselytize; indeed, where possible, they avoid contact with other cultures. However, we must also bear in mind, that Western science is mainly concerned with fighting and preventing disease and has no respect for a medical system which patently neglects to do so. For instance, even very recently in Tibet, the milk of animals with suppurating ulcers was quite fearlessly used – tinged with blood – for making butter. Moreover, not long ago in some parts of Kham in Eastern Tibet, a large percentage of the population still showed blatant signs of serious skin diseases.

This strange co-existence of healing potential and neglect of disease is partly due to the singular attitude of many Asians towards the problem of curing and preventing disease. According to traditional thinking, diseases are not only the result of an incorrect lifestyle, diet and so forth; they are even more often due mainly to 'unhealthy thinking'. Furthermore, diseases, usually only those of a serious nature, are seen as the consequence of errors committed in thought, word and deed during previous lives on earth: a sort of inherited or 'original sin'. Methods which aim at removing only the outward symptoms of disease, strike the Tibetan doctor as superficial. To his way of thinking, a lasting cure can only be effected when the whole mental and emotional world of the patient is taken into account. The possibilities of curing the so-called sufferings of 'fate'[1] however, remain intrinsically problematic, even in the hands of the best doctors.

Regarding the causes of disease, modern medicine is developing towards a greater acceptance of the idea that many afflictions are the product of the psyche; an idea maintained, for instance, by classical Greek medicine. One need only mention the observation of the famous doctor Sir William Osler, that the fate of the consumptive primarily depends on what takes place in his head rather than in his chest. The scope of psychogenetic diseases is continually expanding. Even the origin of chronic joint diseases and crippling forms of arthritis (*arthritis deformans*) can be traced back to extreme reserve, pride and emotional suppression; the 'rigid' condition of the joints is said to be a reflection of the patient's whole mental and emotional attitude. Thus contemporary Western medicine is gravitating towards Tibetan medical views concerning etiology.

Despite the great variety of medical philosophies, it is surprising how often opinions converge, especially in the case of great doctors: Paracelsus' most important concepts, for instance, are somewhat related to the core of

---

[1] *Karma*. Man's fate is not seen as imposed from without, but rather as something he creates himself. (Tr.)

Tibetan and ancient Indian medical teachings. In both cases the 'Life Force' is divided into three essential parts : the 'Intelligence of Nature', the 'Energy of Nature' and 'Inert Matter'. *This 'Three in One' is the fundamental principle of the macrocosm and its microcosmic counterpart, man.* Analytical linear thinking, emphasizing the polarity of opposites, which has been intensified by the age of technology, draws man increasingly away from natural thinking which envisions the world and man in terms of the 'Three'. This makes it extremely difficult for the Westerner to grasp the mental imagery of older cultures, such as that of the tradition-oriented Asian, to which the Tibetan healer belongs.

As already mentioned, in the Tibetan healer's view the causation of disease lies in the 'external' area of disturbance, the 'intermediate' area of mistaken or sinful thinking, or the 'inner' area of 'destiny' or *karma* connected with the religious sphere. Sometimes the cause of a disease is to be found in more than one of these three areas. In by far the majority of cases, the outbreak of a disease results from (1) an imbalance and disharmonious interaction between the three humours, brought about by one or more of the above-mentioned causes, or (2) the so-called 'demonic influences', which are the special subject of the chapter on psychiatry. The precipitating causes also frequently overlap : humoral imbalance facilitates access by 'demonic influences' and on the other hand the latter produce harmful proportions of humours.

The Humours

The 'humours', or fluids are generally distinguished in Tibetan medicine by the designations 'bile', 'air' and 'phlegm'.

The meaning of 'bile' in Tibetan humoral pathology is not the substance known to us as bile, but the subtle principle which is its equivalent. The same applies to 'air' and 'phlegm'. (Also when Paracelsus, for example, speaks of salt, sulphur and quicksilver, he does not mean material salt, sulphur and quicksilver, but rather what these three substances symbolise: the 'soluble', the 'combustible' and the 'fluid'.)

According to ancient Indian medical philosophy, upon which Tibetan healers have drawn substantially, 'air', 'bile' and 'phlegm' correspond to the three principles of mind, energy and inert matter. The long philosophical dissertations on the nature of the three 'humours' or 'principles' (mainly in translation from Sanskrit) are formulated in such a way that even to render them partially intelligible requires tremendous effort. This is firstly because our Western languages rarely contain expressions which lend themselves to a clear representation of these subtleties; and secondly because the Asian healer's nonlinear thinking process, as we may call it, is strongly in evidence in these treatises. This distinctive feature is probably familiar to those who have been involved with the spiritual life of Asia or the Tibetan language for a long time. The same applies to Sanskrit experts, especially those who have compared Sanskrit texts on humoral pathology in leading ancient Indian medical works with Western translations of them (Susruta, Charaka, etc.).

The dominant characteristics of the three humours are adjudged as follows: air is dry and light, bile is hot and phlegm is cold, viscous and heavy. The production of air is encouraged by: spiritual development of the individual (this includes both positive and negative spiritualisation – manifested for example in pride, the subordination of spiritual realisations to material ends and so on); certain activities analogous to spiritual development such as fasting and ascetic practices in general; the violent repression of sexual desire, staying up late at night; the deliberate withholding of the body's natural eliminative processes – urine, faeces, nasal mucus and so forth. The main element in the production of bile is *she-dang*, a term sometimes loosely translated 'hate'. An approximation of its real meaning however, is 'any kind of emotional agitation connected with a person's awareness of himself as an individual'. Excessive activity, ambition or anger and, on the physical level, consumption of alcohol and sexual indulgence, all encourage an increase in bile. One of the chief causes of excessive phlegm is the affected person's lack of insight into man's higher calling and purpose in life (i.e. to ignorance in the spiritual sense). It may also be due to too strong a reliance on a life of comfort and indolence, too strong a reliance on material well-being, sleep during the day and so forth.

In a completely *healthy* person the three humours are harmoniously balanced. They mutually stimulate and equalise each other in perfect accord : phlegm cools bile, bile imparts the appropriate warmth to phlegm, air loosens both the other humours without rousing them too much, and so on.

It is important, moreover, for the maintenance of health, that the entire energy system of the human organism is aligned with the course of the 'great whole'; in other words, that the human microcosm is in stable harmony with the greater order of the macrocosm.[2]

[2] These important interrelations, which the Chinese healing art stresses constantly, albeit in a somewhat different form, play a large part in Tibetan medical philosophy. A detailed description is to be found in P. Cyrill von Korvin-Krasinki's excellent book on Tibetan medicine-philosophy (*Tibetische Medizinphilosophie*, Origo Verlag, Zürich 1953).

Diseases can arise exclusively from this lack of harmony between the macrocosm and the human microcosm. One of the simplest examples is a diet inadequately adapted to the seasonal rhythm which necessitates a variation in the consumption of fat, a larger intake of fruit during autumn and so on. In this respect the Tibetans are, for obvious reasons, less fortunate than the inhabitants of most other parts of the world. It is not rare therefore for the Tibetan physician to have to take a different course of action to establish an equilibrium. This, however, is relatively straightforward and easy to accomplish by, for instance, adjusting the air supply to the seasonal cycle. Excess of air is held to be particularly harmful in summer, which is why more people are inclined to suffer from air ebullitions at this time of year. The tendency of many Westerners, for example, to take off more clothes than usual during summer, is considered a mistake by Tibetans.

'Ebullition' of the Humours

Even though this analogy does not quite hit the nail on the head, the 'ebullition' of a humour might best be compared to food which has become moist and swells up; it then overflows into the domains of the other humours and thereby sets up disturbances. According to different central Asian medical works, the main 'seat' of bile is found in the centre of the body; that of phlegm in its upper part, and that of air in the lower part. In practice, however, each individual humour permeates outwards from its seat to the most diverse regions of the body.

The modern Westerner is, in the majority of cases, more susceptible to the dangers of an excess of bile and/or phlegm than of air. The ancient Indian, on the other hand, leaned towards spiritualisation and meditation and was most exposed to the dangers of increases in air. (Moreover he often tended to let his spirituality slip down into the sphere of sexual indulgence contributing to the ebullition of air, and, in addition, suffered from dietary deficiencies caused partly by food shortage and so on.) In fact the frequency of air diseases in Tibeto-Lamaist medicine, modelled as it is to a large extent on ancient Indian tenets, encompasses an extraordinarily wide area, and this is reflected in Tibetan pharmacology. Amongst the materia medica of central Asia which I came across over the years, approximately sixty per cent, a disproportionately high percentage, are predominantly used in Tibet for combating illnesses caused either wholly or partly by an excess of air. Consequently, in considering Tibetan healing methods, it becomes necessary to adjust certain postulations, which apply to people who are primarily threatened by the dangers of air, to the requirements of Western man who, by virtue of his natural disposition and living conditions, tends to suffer more from phlegm or bile complaints.

The simplicity of the scheme of the three fluids or humours encounters great difficulties in its practical application. Even when the main cause of suffering lies in the ebullition of one particular humour, it often happens that as a result of this general ebullition, another humour becomes disordered locally. Hence the doctor's treatment in a number of cases must be directed towards one humour on the general level, but a completely different one locally.

Let us take a simple example: through negligence or the enforced restraint of his excretory processes, or through continual, serious dietary errors, an individual has contracted the ebullition of air. An excess of air in the digestive organs causes a slowing down, and sometimes even an almost total stoppage of digestive activity. The first humour which, in Tibetan opinion, influences the digestive processes in the stomach is phlegm. Since, when there is no apparent general disturbance of phlegm, its production continues as usual, a very uncomfortable phlegm blockage soon develops in the afflicted person's stomach, which can cause, amongst other things, nausea and headaches. In this instance a good doctor must recognise that a local excess of phlegm indeed exists, but that the real cause of illness lies in a general ebullition of the air humour. He will therefore direct his local treatment to the correction of the phlegm overflow, primarily by administering emetics, after thoroughly preparing the patient as is required in Tibetan medicine. Simultaneously, however, he will carry out a general treatment aimed at eliminating the air excess in the organism as a whole, for example rubbing ointments into the patient's skin, heating the top of his head and curbing the overall production of air.

Without going into too much detail in this glance at the Tibetan art of healing, I would like to include the observation here, that rheumatism, which is the cause of much concern to Western researchers, belongs to a category of diseases in Tibetan medicine parallel to the above. This is because rheumatism is produced by the ebullition of one humour on the general level, but the affected organs are afflicted by the localised, secondary action of another humour. Asthma is also said to belong to a similar category.

Certain ebullitions are likely to attack specific organs. For instance: excessive consumption of onions and garlic –especially when partially sprouted – can cause an ebullition of air, which then rouses bile and harms the fine blood vessels of the eyes.

In the first place, therefore, the healer will endeavour to stem the excessive air excitation. He does this primarily by having the patient wrapped in impermeable blankets at night, and also protected from the fresh air in order to quell the influx of its subtle counterpart, namely *prana*. Besides this, he will employ other methods, such as those already mentioned, to curb air production; he will also encourage a cure of the diseased eyes by treating them with medicinal bandages, liniments and so forth.

Recently, a Western doctor who was suffering from a chronic cough, which had hitherto defied curative attempts of all kinds, asked me what a Tibetan doctor would do in his case. I answered that in the first place he would ascertain, by methods similar to those used in the West to diagnose psychosomatic ailments, whether the cough were not in the final analysis attributable to psychic causes, in spite of all indications to the contrary. In a case like this, even when a well-educated patient and those treating him were quite convinced that it were not so, the cause might still be a psychic one. Should a Tibetan doctor, however, also come to the conclusion that the chronic cough under consideration was not psychological in origin, then two methods of healing would be considered: (1) the searing of, in this case, fifteen different precisely defined points on the surface of the patient's skin, and (2) the administration of curative substances, which, however, are so numerous in this particular case, that the nature of the general and local distribution of humours would first have to be established from diagnostic methods described elsewhere in this book. Only then would it be possible to select the appropriate medicines amongst the many different ones available for this condition.

Tibetan medical literature also deals with so-called secret aspects of the humours. Descriptions of them are sym-

bolic to the extent that literal translations are almost
grotesque and have been used on occasion to try to dis-
credit and ridicule the entire outlook and spiritual life[3]
of the Tibetans. Some attempts to open up spiritual realms
with the scalpel of analytical reasoning, are very reminiscent of the unimaginative Inca scholar, who studied Chris-
tianity at the time of the Spanish conquest of South
America at the behest of the Inca authorities. In doing so
he came to the following 'learned' and 'logical' conclu-
sions: 'The Christians believe in one God. However, they
also believe in three divinities. That makes, therefore, a
total of four.'

In harmony with the course run by the macrocosm, the
humours are also subject to a daily and a seasonal rhythm
of increase and decrease, which good Tibetan doctors take
into account in their fight against the ebullition of humours. Hence phlegm, for example, is strongest during winter and the first half of spring. Phlegm *per se* is also supposed to be more prevalent during the night, so that
people who suffer from an excess of phlegm usually experience greater distress at night than in the daytime.

'Hot' and 'Cold' Diseases

In addition to the general category of disturbances produced by the various humours, there are further subdivisions into 'hot' and 'cold'. The direct cause of 'hot' diseases is said to be bile and/or 'ebullition of hot blood',
which results in the disharmony of all three humours;
whilst most 'cold' diseases are said to be the product of

[3] German: Geistesleben. "Geist" means both mind or intellect and
spirit or soul, amongst other things. The exact connotation of this
word is vague. In the first centuries A.D. Westerners considered man
as an aggregate of body, soul and spirit, but much later this was
changed to a dualistic concept of body plus soul.

'phlegm' ebullitions. The 'seat' of illnesses originating primarily in the disharmony of several humours, can apparently most often be found in and around four organs, namely : the stomach, the liver, the 'upper part' of the intestine, or 'its lower part'. (Tibetan terminology makes a distinction by means of these two expressions.)

According to a detailed description in the *len-thab*, a noted medical work, air diseases fall into no less than twenty different groups, the division of which is not always according to organs. In hot air diseases, disturbances are already combined with additional ebullitions of bile during the first stage, whereas in cold ones both air and phlegm have begun to malfunction during the first stage, even though in both cases there is predominant air ebullition. Symptoms which accompany air diseases include dizziness, trembling, ringing in the ears, a dry tongue, excessive yawning, a jumpy heart-beat, also sleeplessness and pains in the back and jaws (as signs of a general disturbance). Each subdivision of air diseases is subject again to its particular symptoms : if the seat is in the head, this is denoted by ringing in the ears and a tendency to vomit. Alcohol should be avoided in hot air diseases. *Chang* beer, usually drunk hot, has an otherwise beneficial effect on air affections, as also do massages – old butter is used as a lubricant – and also a diet of some kinds of meat.

In this connection, experts on central Asia will probably be surprised that the Tibetan doctor prescribes meat and beer without concern for the religious precepts of Lamaism. In practice the Tibetan is little inclined towards fanaticism and the observation of any kind of absolute rules or precepts. He knows all too well that, depending on the circumstances, any limitation whatever can be destructive as well as beneficial.

Not only phlegm but air too can provoke a general uprising of the other humours. The afore-mentioned medical work says with regard to this, that air can function like bellows, which, as it were, 'kindles' the other humours – many Tibetan authors love vivid metaphors!

The same work designates bile affections as generally very difficult to cure. In fact, it says, there are no less than forty-seven different bile diseases which are, nevertheless, quite easy to divide into hot and cold. One of the most significant symptoms of hot bile diseases is said to be a continuous, almost unquenchable thirst; of cold ones, perpetual digestive disturbances.

An excessively large, frequent or irregular food intake and damp bedclothes are reckoned amongst the causes of phlegm ebullitions.

Diagnostic procedure is extremely simple. 'Thick' urine signifies an excess of bile; if it is yellowish-red a hot bile disease is indicated. Very frothy urine points to an excess of air, and when completely odourless, to phlegm. A thick, yellowish fur on the tongue is an indication of bile, a rough, dry tongue of air, and a thin, whitish fur of phlegm.

It is only after studying the standard medical literature in depth, that one begins to realise the infinite complications involved in the practical application of the whole doctrine. It is not surprising then, to learn that before the Tibetan doctor is taken seriously as a healing practitioner he must train for up to twenty years.

The mutual relationship between macrocosm and microcosm, and the acknowledgement of karmic or pre-destined suffering, force the doctor to take into account each time deeper and more complex interconnections in his calculations. This is because using medicines and various treatment methods to 'hold back' the humours in their natural given areas, and reconstitute them to harmonious proportions, can only bring about a temporary improvement; and indeed, in the case of unskilled or too technically-minded healers, can even cause the trouble simply to shift from one organ to another.

One of the chief concerns, especially of the most devoted healers, is to prevent exploitation of their knowledge by the unworthy. The profane category of people includes those of a certain character and personality – equipped with only a certain amount of learning – who are what the Tibetan language of letters refers to as 'inferior human vessels'.

Lamaist medicine, and also the Chinese traditional art of healing, has an ideal image of the healer. He is not only reckoned in every respect a man of noble character, but he is also capable of immediately making the right diagnosis of a patient's illness, without any examination or the least assistance. He is looked upon as selfless and wise; the epitome of the pure man. Every genuine central Asian healer admits that people of such calibre are exceptionally rare.

The Pulse Diagnosis

Healers who use intricate diagnostic methods in order to establish the nature of a disease – in other words the large majority of Asian healing practitioners – are ranked by Tibeto-Lamaist medicine, and by ancient Chinese medicine too, amongst the fourth and lowest category of their healers. Perhaps one of the most important of their aids is the pulse diagnosis.

Within the diagnostic context, a 'full' pulse is an indication of a general over-abundance of bile, a 'jumpy' one of air, and a 'sluggish and heavy' one of phlegm.

Tibetan medicine distinguishes eleven types of pulse, in

contrast to the traditional Chinese school which recognises about two hundred. The foundations of Lamaist medicine go back to ancient Indian models for the most part, but it would appear that with respect to the pulse diagnosis they were inspired by the Chinese example, albeit with considerable simplifications. Amongst the two hundred types of pulse in traditional Chinese medicine, one finds unsteady, deep, slippery, sluggish, strong, coarse, fluctuating, hollow, rapid, missing, wide, tremulous, amplified, dilated, average and so on. With the additional variations and complications related to different daily and seasonal rhythms, the patient's bodily constitution and so forth, the Chinese doctor arrives at the said two hundred types of pulse.[4]

The famous physician Pien-chueh (fifth century B.C.) discovered the diagnostic significance of the pulse. His important discovery only reached the West many centuries later by a very roundabout route via the Arab world. Traditional Chinese medicine distinguishes three pulse zones of roughly the width of a finger on each wrist. The area of the right pulse nearest the fingers corresponds to the lungs, that of the left to the heart, the right middle section to the stomach and spleen, and the left middle section to the gall-bladder and liver. The area on the right wrist nearest the shoulder corresponds to the large intestine and kidneys, and on the left to the small intestine and urinary bladder. The pulses should be taken early in the morning, since it is at this time that their characteristics stand out most clearly. A skilled Asian healer should be able to ascertain very quickly from palpation of the pulse zones which of the patient's organs is diseased.

The Tibetan doctor's pulse examination is similar to

---

[4] These also include superficial and deep pulses. (Translator)

that in traditional Chinese medicine: he usually palpates the patient's entire pulse area with his three middle fingers. In some cases, however, examination of the pulse also extends to the chief arteries in other areas of the body, especially the temples.

When the ordinary Tibetan doctor, whose status roughly equals that of the fourth grade in Chinese medicine, is called to a patient, he usually begins by putting twenty-nine questions to him, prescribed by standard medical works in the 'Forbidden Land' for this situation. They concern the types of pains and complaints caused by the disease, the effects of the most important foods last consumed by the sick person, the general circumstances of his life, his sex life and so forth. Only then does he proceed to examine the tongue, urine and pulse.

Interpretation of Dreams

Many healers also attribute importance to the interpretation of dreams. According to the chapter entitled *mi-lam-mi-pe-zang-ngen* in the Tibetan work *kun-dzon-ya-sel-me-long* for instance, dreams about wearing new clothes and headgear for the first time, or singing in the mountain tops, of sunrise and riding good horses, are all positive signs for the course of the disease. Dreaming of corals, being followed by malevolent animals, digging holes in the ground and cutting down shrubs (as is well known, there are no trees throughout most of Tibet) are, on the other hand, considered decidedly unfavourable signs for the further development of a disease. The same text considers dreams in which the patient is sitting naked, wandering around disoriented in desert regions, picking red flowers and climbing in wild mountainous regions, as dangerous signs of a fatal disease.

Further passages, evidently translated from the Sanskrit

and the Chinese, lay down an exact dream-diagnosis related to organs. According to them, dreaming of over-tiredness and swimming against strong, dangerous currents is regarded as a sign of kidney malfunction; dreaming about streams and waterfalls a symptom of anaemia; of wandering around desolate mountain tops, which are difficult regions to traverse, and about grass and bushes, as a sign of liver malfunction.

The Tibetan scientist of distinction, however, regards this sort of dream-diagnosis as too primitive. In his opinion, it is the symbolic significance of a dream as a whole, as interpreted within a much larger context, which yields deeper diagnostic implications, rather than an analysis of its content in terms of objects and so forth.

Eye-diagnosis is well known to a section of the Tibetan medical profession. In contrast to Western practices (of iridiagnosis[5]), however, it is based on a thorough examination of the pupil. It is, of course, much more difficult to identify irregularities in different zones of the pupil than the iris.

Particularly important with regard to diagnosis is the fact that sometimes the Tibetan doctor cannot make an absolutely definite diagnosis, even on the basis of a group of symptoms which seem as good as conclusive. This requires further explanation. For another very important difference between Tibetan and Western medicine is that, according to Tibetan belief, there exists an 'intermediate world' between the world of pure spirit and that of gross materiality. It is said to permeate the latter and only because of this can an actual interaction take place between spirit and matter. One aspect of this intermediate world is the 'second body'.

[5] Translator

The Second Body

IN VIEW OF the continuous interaction between the second body and the dense material human body, the Tibetan doctor will only very unwillingly and in the most extreme emergencies turn to surgical instruments. (He does, of course, also realise only too well how relatively primitive his operating methods are. These are the subject of a later chapter.) As a general rule, however, he does not believe that one should operate on diseased parts of the body without also working simultaneously on their subtle counterparts.

The second body, this subtle counterpart of the coarse body-husk, is said to be permeated by thousands of channels of varying density.[1] Many Tibetan healers reckon their sum total to be in the region of one hundred thousand. Various written and oral references made by central Asian doctors suggest that many, or even the great majority, of these channels are so arranged that their paths coincide with those of many blood vessels and nerve fibres, in that they follow the same course, often winding themselves around them. This could also be the reason why so many Asian healing practitioners tend to designate blood vessels and nerves by the same terms. They are

[1] Cf. Govinda *Foundations of Tibetan Mysticism*, ed. Rider & Co., part 4, chapter 5. (Translator)

probably thinking first and foremost of these 'conductors', and in the light of this concept dense material manifestations fade into the background. We have only to glance at the history of Western medicine, by the way, to encounter similar ideas. For many hundreds of years before Galen it was believed that the blood vessels in man contained 'air'. Galen was described as the first to discover that this is not so. How can one insult the entire medical profession of times past, who have excelled themselves in many respects, by taking them for simpletons who during the course of centuries had not noticed that blood vessels contain blood? Is it not more likely that they, like the Asian medical profession, when speaking of 'air' in this context, had a subtle counterpart in mind?

The channels of the second body – which, similar to visible blood vessels, vary widely in order of magnitude – serve to circulate the subtle counterpart of air. (This circulatory system is not to be confused with that of the seat of vitality or life force, which is discussed later.) According to Tibetan medicine, many diseases, like asthma for instance, arise by dint of subtle air dragging along subtle phlegm, which then blocks the channels. One discovers that Hippocrates also had similar ideas, if one reads him observantly. In doing so, it should not be forgotten that here too, modern translators face an awkward problem : they have to translate expressions for processes which lie beyond the scope of the gross material plane, by terms which can only with difficulty convey the essence of such subtleties. If, for instance, one reads the translation of Hippocrates' description of epilepsy,[2] one cannot avoid having the feeling that the expression 'vena cava' mentioned in it, is not really to be taken literally.

[2] Hippocrates, *De la Maladie Sacrée, Oeuvres Complètes*, éd. et trad. Littré, tome VI, p. 367. (Translator)

The circulation of subtle air through the channels is, so to speak, the counterpart of the circulation of the blood, breathing and neural activity. It is apparently only at this level, that the mutual relationship between the three comes fully into play. Certain contradictions, therefore, which result when these three important functions are viewed exclusively in gross material terms, are clarified when seen in this light. Methods of influencing this 'circulation' are possible and include breathing exercises, especially ones combined with certain mental exercises in concentration. These can be dangerous, however, since everyone apparently has his own personal breathing rhythm, which is peculiar to him alone and suited to his entire being as a man endowed with spirit existing on the material plane. Hence, this type of curative technique runs the risk of gaining tangible results at the cost of very subtle spiritual damage. Above all, brusque changes in breathing rhythm are warned against.

Breathing exercises in the 'Forbidden Land' should, as a rule, only be practised under the watchful eye of a teacher specially called to the task, who nearly always has many years of experience to draw on. Whether one can even contemplate such practices for the West is very difficult to answer, since it is in subtle spheres of precisely this nature that the Westerner may react differently from the Tibetan. In the first place, various meditation and trance states[3] and the Tibetan breathing exercises combined with them, *lung-gom*, seem to require the total freedom of the individual from nervous excitability in the Western sense. So it is doubtful at the outset, whether many Westerners would be possible candidates for such practices.

[3] The term for 'trance' in Tibetan does not, by the way, mean quite the same as it does in the West. The Tibetan seems to be far less passive in most of his trance states than is the case in those induced in the West.

The three largest channels are called *ro-ma, u-ma* and *kyang-ma* and are said to wind themselves 'corkscrew-fashion' around the spinal column. In doing so, they only meet at two points, namely at their root or base situated near the coccyx and at their upper end in the region of the crown of the head.[4] The dense human body seems to be most closely connected with the second body in the area of the spine. The central Asian physician is therefore of the opinion that here, especially, any operations which fail to take account of the subtle equivalents are most dangerous. In relation to this, I recall a commentary by an Asian scholar who, in spite of his enormous tolerance with respect to other issues, could hardly conceal his absolute horror after hearing a detailed account of our modern pneumo-encephalography in the West.

It is a remarkable fact that in moxa or moxibustion – the burning of aromatic herbs over certain points of the skin surface, which is discussed in the chapter on curative methods – the points in question coincide with places that seem to correspond with the anatomy of the subtle channels. This is probably also the case with acupuncture points; in other words, it could be that this too is a matter of directly influencing the second body. It is therefore no wonder that material oriented research has not succeeded in finding any obvious, logical reasons for the efficacy of moxa and acupuncture.[5]

The three main channels in the second body course upwards from below. A powerful mass of latent 'cosmic

[4] Opinions vary concerning this subtle anatomy. Cf. Govinda *Foundations of Tibetan Mysticism*, p. 146, and Evans-Wentz *Tibetan Yoga and Secret Doctrines*, p. 157. (Translator)

[5] The existence of the second body and its relation to acupuncture are the subject of statements by L. Schroeder and S. Ostrander *Psychic Discoveries Behind the Iron Curtain*, ch. 18. (Translator)

energy' condensed into a very small space is said to be located in their lowest part. The more someone aligns his life with a higher order in the truly religious sense – in other words, lives his whole life as a single thanksgiving to creation, instead of placing demands on it – the more these forces begin to unfold of themselves.

It is reported that the usual consequence of using artificial methods to release these forces is that the person concerned fails to control the energies thus liberated, and they often become converted into 'animal dynamism' when still in the lower part of the main channels. In mild cases this can supposedly lead to severe damage to health; in serious ones, however, to insanity, or else it can lay the foundations for the still more frightening spiritual catastrophe discussed later in the chapter on psychiatry. This is said to be one of the most important reasons why much of the knowledge concerning various aspects of the second body ought to continue to be protected in the form of secret teachings.

Several books published in recent years contain outlines in varying detail of the seven vital energy centres situated on the three primary channels. These centres are known as *chakra* in ancient Indian medicine and in Tibeto-Lamaist medicine as *khorlo*. According to the Central Asian sage, the information disclosed in such expositions goes to the utmost limit that the average person today can take without – as they put it – 'being tempted to destroy himself'.

The Lamaist doctor has a wide range of remedial techniques at his disposal. In addition to his medicaments, which are the subject of a later chapter, massage is one of the methods of treatment which can affect not only the gross material human body, but also its subtle counterpart. This massage does not just consist of a simple knead-ing in the customary sense. It is rather a manipulation of the body by the healer's hands, which are charged with *prana*. Amongst high ranking healers, this is combined with corresponding mental images, *migpa*. I have observed such massages and I noticed that, for practical purposes, the strokes can be divided into two different categories: circular and lengthwise. The one seems to charge the or-ganism with subtle, non-material energies and the other to discharge them. The kneading works simultaneously on the gross material body and produces amongst other things, the dissipation of phlegm blockages.

To the limited number of observers of essential facets of central Asian life belongs A. de Reincourt. When asked to what extent an individual may use his psychic powers in the 'Forbidden Land', he gave the following reply: 'There is a difference between those who are equipped with psychic powers from their earliest youth, and the Lamas who cultivate such powers through meditation exercises and arduous training. Only the former, who usually possess these powers at the cost of severe physical handicaps, may utilise them. Psychic powers acquired by personal effort should not be used for the attainment of worldly objectives'.

Exceptions will of course arise, primarily when the doctor is quite convinced that the sick person intends to devote himself to a life of creative activity, once his health is restored. Resolving this question may well be fraught with some pangs of conscience for healers with a sense of their responsibility. Indeed, the Tibetan sage sees these conflicts as constituting part of the plans of a higher order, which forces every creature to make inde-pendent decisions commensurate with his spiritual level, whereby each becomes, as it were, 'his own judge'. In any case, it is considered customary in Tibet to proffer an especially high recompense to a healer who, to effect a cure, gives a portion of his own life force to the patient, over and above using ordinary curative methods.

All in all, the second body is in a much more unstable position than the dense human body. It is said to adjust itself with lightning speed to each and every shift in a person's mental and emotional worlds. The vitality of the double body – and its centre too – are subject to constant change. This centre of vitality changes and shifts its position according to a specific daily and monthly rhythm. Many Tibetan healing practitioners attribute great significance to the latter particularly.

It is not easy to determine a precise equivalent of the Tibetan second body from amongst the designations used by Western occultists. Many believe in an aggregate of such intermediate bodies, with varying degrees of subtle density. Moreover, many branches of occultism even disagree as to what exactly the so-called 'astral body' is and how they should define it. When a Tibetan healer distinguishes between the subtle counterparts of the gross material organism, he usually tends to do so in terms of function.

Physicians of higher standing – that is those whose spiritual level roughly corresponds to the highest category in ancient China – are said to be able actually to perceive the second body, beyond the perceptual capacity of the sense organs. In doing so, equivalents of the gross material organs apparently come into play on other levels.[6]

---

[6] Photographs have been taken of the energy allegedly emitted by the intermediate world. The matter is still controversial. Cf. *Psychic Discoveries Behind the Iron Curtain*. (Translator)

The colours of a healthy second body are described as intensely brilliant. Its colourful splendour is subject to constant changes corresponding to shifts in the mental and emotional states of the person concerned. A state of ill-health can apparently often be distinguished by a dark and gloomy array of colours.

People of a pure nature and on a high spiritual level are said to have particularly striking and beautiful second bodies, which extend much further beyond the periphery of the dense physical body than those of average people. In such cases the second body is supposed to emanate unusually bright rays of light, notably in the area of the head and hands.

In the relationship between the gross body and its subtle counterpart, neither one takes the dominant role. The second body is said to be nourished, as it were, by the subtle essence of food. In certain trance states it can apparently nourish itself without the additional help of the body, by absorbing subtle materials directly from the environment. This is also said to be possible in a normal state for people specially endowed, who are at a particularly high stage of spiritual development. They are however rare exceptions. It is also generally admitted that the number of healers who can actually perceive the second body is extremely limited.

In Tibetan literature, direct perception of the subtle equivalents of the three humours in the second body is very rarely discussed, least of all when it concerns their so-called secret counterparts.

In trance states, during sleep and so on, the larger part of the dense body's subtle counterpart is said to withdraw from it temporarily. It remains connected to it, however, by means of a sort of invisible thread. This is the state in which so-called 'demonic influences' – the main subject of the chapter on psychiatry – can take effect most easily. Clairvoyant healers are in a position, it seems, to perceive how such external forces take a grip on the aura, discolour it, darken it, infiltrate it and so on. Incantations influence this subtle body, in so far as the individuals who utter them are capable of causing the outgoing vibration, as it is called, to communicate its oscillations to other levels. I had an opportunity, together with several others, to observe how Asian healers uttered their incantations in a closed room so that the walls began to vibrate, so to speak, together with part of the interior decor. In instances involving eminent healers, the area of vibration can extend so far that it simultaneously reaches and affects the subtle regions of the second body.

The seat of the life force in the second body is said to be in the sole of the right foot on the first day of the Tibetan month. (A Tibetan month always lasts thirty days. The year has twelve months. From time to time entire intercalary months are inserted to match up with the astronomical calendar.) The centre of life force climbs upwards along the right foot and reaches the thigh on the sixth day; then up along the right half of the body to the right shoulder on the tenth day. From here it proceeds up the right side of the head towards the top and reaches the right cheek on the fourteenth day. Once it has reached the crown of the head on the fifteenth day, it disperses itself throughout the entire body for a short time. It then courses down the left side of the body at the same speed during the next fifteen days. On the thirtieth day it reaches the sole of the left foot and disperses itself throughout the entire body again for a short while. On the first day of the following month it begins a fresh cycle starting out from the sole of the right foot.

In women the seat of vitality circulates in the opposite

direction and begins in the sole of the left foot.

I include the observation here, not to be overlooked, that this cycle is not considered completely authoritative in Tibet; indeed, I myself found divergent descriptions.

Tibetan Medical Writings

THE ORIGIN of the Tibetan language has not been satisfactorily clarified. We know from the script alone that it was created about eleven hundred years ago, under the auspices of an important ruler who was a Buddhist convert; that it was based on an ancient Indian syllabic script; and that the transition to the present script occurred with the adoption of Buddhism. A fusion of cultures took place: very old indigenous and traditional elements coalesced with Buddhism as it filtered in from India. This process of amalgamation also included medicine. In addition, the Tibetan healing art has, in the course of time, adopted parts of traditional Chinese medicine and integrated them extensively into its theory and practice.

Medical literature is copious. Although Tibetan 'universities' are divided into four faculties, one of which is medical, the borderline between medical and non-medical writings is much less clear than in the West. Alongside books which are unequivocally medical in content, there are many which also deal with medical matters within a distinctly non-medical framework. Thus it is often not easy to recognise them immediately, even for someone well acquainted with the language and literature. Besides this, the titles of Tibetan works do not always give an accurate reflection of their contents.

Books usually consist of loose, horizontal-oblong leaves, printed or written on both sides, which – particularly in the case of more highly valued manuscripts – are wrapped in a piece of cloth called *nam-za*, and sometimes kept between two hard covers. The leaves are not always numbered. It can happen that at the beginning of a new leaf, one suddenly notices that the text is on a different spiritual level and in a different style. Obviously, part of the content has been substituted in such cases by different texts, which look very similar on the surface. I was once invited to look through some privately owned, rare Tibetan manuscripts, because the owners wanted to know something concerning their content. The manuscript delved more and more deeply into so-called secret domains, until it finally came to a page in which many passages were heavily crossed out so as to make them illegible. From the next page on, the manuscript was once again very neat and clear, but on a completely different spiritual level. Apparently part of the content had been substituted by pages which seemed similar outwardly, in order to avoid a public display of the more important part of the manuscript, but without arousing the reader's curiosity by the obvious omission.

Tibetan writings rarely contain even a remotely systematic enumeration of chapters or their contents. In the case of the *gyu-shi*, for example, a very comprehensive Lamaist work consisting of more than one hundred and sixty sections, this is a hindrance which is sufficient in itself to impede exploitation by persons who might misuse the knowledge gained.

By far the majority of Tibetan books and manuscripts are drafted either in the printing characters called *u-chen* or in the learned characters called *u-me*. Although the latter is less common and even better suited to veiling the content than the former, far from all secret texts are drafted in this learned script. Knowledge of it has, moreover, spread greatly during recent years, and it is taught today in the schools of the capital.[1]

The scrupulousness mentioned earlier, with which the content of texts is concealed from exploiters motivated by considerations of worldly profit, is remarkable. Quite apart from the camouflaging and the symbolism of the afore-mentioned 'inner' and 'secret' spheres, they seem to harbour such a great fear of people of inferior character, that they take at least precautionary measures, even in the case of straightforward descriptive texts. These measures enable only those who have engaged in intensive studies of the Tibetan language for many years to grasp the contents. An exploiter of a so-called practical turn of mind would obviously be unlikely to have either the time or the inclination to do this, since, whichever way you go about it, long years of study are involved! In the same way, they take additional precautions with printed secret manuscripts – like the above-mentioned *gyu-shi* – which consist of either omitting the dots at the end of syllables; or rendering them almost illegible; or alternatively putting them quite deliberately in the wrong place, in order to mislead all those who would decipher the texts in pursuit of personal gain.

The absence of lucid arrangement in Tibetan medical literature makes the verification of quoted passages much more difficult than in the West. Nevertheless, the situation is less chaotic than one would initially imagine. Tibetan healers know many stretches of the standard

[1] This was written in 1957, before the Chinese occupation. We do not know if it is taught under the Communist régime. (Tr.)

medical works by heart, and they can often see immediately whether references to other medical writings make
sense in a larger context. Furthermore, it is easier in Tibetan works than in the writings of other cultures to recognise the intellectual stature of an author and to assess him
correctly, even when it is not possible to follow up his
references to other medical works. However remarkable
it may sound, especially for a country where the oppor-
tunities to plagiarize with impunity are far greater than
elsewhere, the preparation of a new book by compiling
passages from extant texts is actually much more difficult.
This is because the new product may fall prey to ridicule
if it does not reflect the living personality of the author
and his individual experience.

Generally speaking, many Asian scholars prefer to regard books and notes primarily as mental supports and
transitional aids, whilst they keep the actual keys in their
heads. This is why, when a healer from central Asia of
Badmajeff's rank was captured during a period of revolu-
tion, and all his notes were examined by interpreters and
an analysis made of his different cures, they were no
wiser than a pair of oxen confronted by a table of loga-
rithms!

Symbolic representations are easier to formulate in
Tibetan writings, because the Tibetan language itself tends
to leave things hanging in the balance. The expression
nang-wa, for instance, means, (1) light, in the ordinary
sense of the word; (2) objects and so forth which become
visible in light; and (3) light in the sense of the inward
appearance of mental pictures.

Even if all the texts were printed clearly and with the
dot in the right place at the end of syllables, the philolo-
gist's scalpel would probably only touch on the superficial
level of meaning and not penetrate the inner symbolic or

even esoteric significance. In a Western rendering of a Tibetan text for instance, the words *yul-tham-che-tong-par-thong-ne* are translated as, 'when he saw all lands desolate'. The word *yul*, however, does not only mean land in the geographical sense, but also sphere of sensory perception, in other words, that which man is able to cognize with his senses. *Tong* means empty, which the translator then adapted to the presumed sense of the word *yul* (land) by desolate. *Thong* does in fact mean to see. The meaning of the above-mentioned quotation is therefore, not, 'when he saw all lands (in the geographical sense) desolate', but, 'when, as far as he was concerned, all objects of external sensory perception had become empty, in other words, had lost their significance'; hence, that he reached a state of consciousness, in which his normal sensory faculties were shut off!

In Tibetan texts the actual, more profound meaning often lies in that which is intentionally left unsaid. An example: in a treatise on practical philosophy one reads, 'Treat your enemies kindly and with forbearance. Thus will you conquer them'. Immediately following this the opposite is stated, 'If you have enemies, conquer them with extreme severity'! The real meaning here is contained in the contradiction between the two consecutive statements. Roughly then, 'Treat your enemies as befits the particular situation'! But this is precisely what remains unformulated!

In those texts which are distinctly esoteric, the symbolism can go so far that even short passages require lengthy reflection. Literal translations produce absolute nonsense.[2]

And the more superior a Tibetan text is, the more it

---

[2] This is, of course, not only peculiar to Tibetan literature. A respected Hindu work describes as follows the 'after death state' of a 'good and somewhat erudite' person:

lacks long discussions and explanations. Important trains of thought and blueprints are the result of a few skilfully employed significant words. The *tsig-nyung-la-don-dye-pa* (roughly : far-reaching [and poignant] characterisations with very few words) is one of the strongest indications of an important Lamaist medical work.

Even material on 'concrete' levels is extraordinarily difficult to understand in Tibetan medical works. Learned authors tend, amongst other things, arbitrarily to abbreviate the longer quotations which they presume their educated readers are familiar with. They do this without guidance of any rules or considerations which are in the least bit logical. It is just as though an English writer were to substitute "To be, or not to be" or "I wandered lonely as a cloud" by the letter sequence 'benobe' and 'waloclou', taking it for granted that the educated reader will understand what these abbreviations mean, without any explanation whatever! Besides this, in many medical, and especially pharmacological texts, metaphors are often used, which are even difficult for many an educated Tibetan to understand. These denote metals, precious stones, frequently used medicinal substances and so forth; such as 'son of the moon' for calcite, or 'eightfooted one' for gold. Even amongst precise designations, the borderlines of meaning are often more blurred than in Western and many other Asian languages. The result is that the same word can mean 'shoulder area', for example, as well as 'upper arm' in medical terminology. Chinese medicine

---

"He steps up to the light; from the light to the day; from the day to the shining side of the half moon; from thence to the six months, during which the sun moves towards the north; from here to the year; from the year to the sun; from the sun to the moon; from the moon to the lightning. There he then meets the being who accompanies him to the highest and most sublime region".

also lets many an ambiguity pass in its literature – obviously on purpose. This is sometimes taken to such an extent, that they use characters which mean 'womb' as well as 'bladder', or 'stomach' as well as 'spleen', without explaining which of the two organs is meant in the case in hand. At all events, it is presumed that someone familiar with medical facts will perceive immediately from the context, which of the two organs is meant.

Even the biggest dictionaries are only of very limited practical value where Tibetan medicine is concerned. One finds, for instance, the same substance featuring in Lamaist materia medica 'translated' in one place by 'gold-leaf', but elsewhere by 'vitriol'. If one pursues the matter with the help of a very comprehensive Tibetan book on pharmacology, for example the *du-tsi-men-dyi-nam-ye-ngo-wo-nu-ming-dye-par-she-pa-dri-me-shel-gong*, one can ascertain that the substance in question is none other than soda!

*

There follows here a list of a number of Tibetan medical works, the contents of which I was mainly considering in writing this book. The rendering of the Tibetan titles basically follows the current[3] pronunciation used by learned Tibetans in that country's capital, which may be regarded as a kind of lingua franca of the 'Forbidden Land'.

Important original Tibetan texts and works translated into Tibetan: the *gyu-shi*; *len-thab*; *kun-dzob-ya-sel-me-long* (especially the chapter on the Tibetan doctor's clinical pictures of disease); the *du-shom-pe-nyem-po-tsi-men-dyi-nu-pa-kyang-she-sel-ton-dri-me-she-pe-dri-me-she-treng*; works by the Tibetan author *mi-pam-jam-pel-dye-pa* (espe-

---

[3] 1957 (Tr.)

cially the passages on Tibetan materia medica); the *Kumara-Tantra* (translated from the Sanskrit); *tso-we-tse-yi-pag-sam-jon* (particularly the chapter on psychiatry); the *Suvarnaprabhasottamasutra* (translated from the Sanskrit); the translations of Chinese medical works: the *Ching-Kuei-Yao-Lue*; the *Huang-Ti-Nei-Ching*; the *Shen-Nung-Pen-Tsao-Ching*; the *Shang-Han-Lun* (section on Tibetan medical writings).

Here are two short extracts from texts. By Tibetan standards these passages are easy to understand!

(1) From the *King of Medical Works*: 'Curative possibilities for disease, infinite number. Without knowledge of healing, like an arrow shot downwards'. Meaning: There are infinite varieties of healing procedures. If, however, one is not capable of choosing the correct healing method from amongst them, one is like someone who shoots an arrow downwards, i.e. in vain.

(2) From the Tibetan translation of the *Suvarnaprabhasottamasutra*: 'Time and not time to eat food in relation good effect. This and that in the human body does not harm the body's fire.' This answers the questions: The effect of food on a person in relation to its timely or untimely consumption? Does it also depend on this food or that whether the 'fire in the body' (this means the 'digestive fire', in other words, the digestive function) is damaged?

In the light of the preceding comments on the peculiarities of Tibetan literature, it should be quite obvious to any discerning person, that the supposition of a well known European scientist interested in turning central Asian medicine to some account, that he could simply rope in some interpreters and, after completing the work of translation, crown himself medical king, is considered an inopportune joke by learned Asians!

Translations into Tibetan also often take account of the spiritual calibre of the original. I once had the opportunity of carefully comparing two different Tibetan translations of the same unusually difficult text, by two obviously highly educated Tibetans, who were not familiar with one another. Both versions were made in Tibet; one of the original texts had arrived there by the – in those times – enormously roundabout route from Eastern China via Mongolia, the other via India. From an objective standpoint, the two translations were so different from each other, that one could barely find one expression that was the same in both, or even vaguely similar. Separately, however, each had grasped the conceptual content of the original on the spiritual level correctly, and given clear expression to it in his own way.

The quantity of medical literature translated into Tibetan is much greater than the number of medical books and manuscripts written in the land itself in the course of time. It incorporates, above all, a great abundance of translations of ancient Indian medical works and also many traditional Chinese ones. Various aspects of the wisdom and experience belonging to the treasury of the ancient Chinese healing art were absorbed into the Tibetan medical system. The former had already reached a high level of development many centuries before our era. At the time of the Tang Dynasty, which roughly coincides with the time when Buddhism penetrated into Tibet (in other words, when the 'Forbidden Land' laid the foundations of its present-day medical science), China was *the* medical centre of Asia. It already had the first proper medical school of international standing, at which many doctors from outside China – Japan, Korea, numerous other Asian countries and part of the Arab world – acquired their medical knowledge.

Tibetan translations from Sanskrit include all the more important works by the most famous ancient Indian doctors – Charaka, Susruta, Vasabandhu and so on. To illustrate an additional point: a few years ago when a German translation from Sanskrit of an important work by Vasubandhu appeared in Holland, and I tried to track down a Tibetan translation of the same work in order to look into the meaning of various unclear points, I discovered that I could obtain one without any trouble from Japan. The original of many Sanskrit medical texts have, incidentally, long since disappeared, but they are available nonetheless in Tibetan translation, either in Tibet or other countries.

Amongst the medical works translated into Tibetan from Chinese, there are not only numerous texts on the theory and practice of pulse diagnosis and other relevant literature, but also a great number of the most important traditional Chinese texts on other aspects of the healing art. Amongst these are Tibetan versions of the *Ching-Kuei-Yao-Lue* on 'important medical facts'; the famous *Huang-Ti-Nei-Ching* (a work composed on the basis of very ancient medical traditions, which was already well known in China in the third century B.C.); the *Shen-Nung-Pen-Tsao-Ching*, concerning the curative effects of three hundred substances, including the use of quicksilver and sulphur in the treatment of skin diseases[4]; the famous *Shang-Han-Lun* on the nature and treatment of fevers; and many others.

The last-mentioned book includes an excellent descrip-

[4] This medical work was already known in the first century B.C. and anticipated by centuries the medical tenets of various cultures.

Incidentally, in Chinese literature it is far easier to ascertain the period in which a work originates than in the Tibetan. The Tibetans

tion of the course of epidemic diseases, including typhus, beginning from the first symptoms, such as loss of appetite, rigor and nose bleed, up to the final stages. Cold baths, which are said to strengthen the patient and diminish delirium, are prescribed for a high fever in typhus. No purgatives are prescribed for this disease. Lamaist medicine, however, because of its overemphasis on the 'demon conditioned' aspect of disease in the sphere of infectious diseases, has certainly fallen behind the ancient Chinese in this particular field.

The integration of traditional Chinese medical tenets into their own philosophy of healing, could not always have been easy for Lamaist doctors. The philosophical background of the Chinese (polarity of *yin* and *yang* and all its ramifications; the ancient Chinese concept of 'occult anatomy'; the entire sphere of traditional Chinese pathology, and so on) differs considerably from many Tibetan concepts. Of course, there are on the other hand many points where they converge on the spiritual level, in their attitude to the patient and so forth. An important precept of the traditional Chinese doctor runs: *pai-wen-pu-ju-yi-chien* ('One look is worth more than a hundred words'). Meaning: even the most thorough study of medical teachings bears no comparison to the experience of visiting a patient once.

A particularly important difference between the modern Western concept of the role of medical literature and

---

reckon according to a sixty year cycle. In nearly every work it is easy to establish in which year of a cycle the book was written. However, there is an absence of any indication as to the relevant *cycle*! Experts on Tibetan literature can distinguish the cycle either from the name of the author (if he was at all well known and the name is not very commonplace); or from certain historical and other contexts; from the style too, as a last resort, from which an expert can draw inferences as to the time when the particular book or manuscript was drafted.

that of the ancient Chinese, is that the tradition-based
Asian healer considers his texts primarily as a *point
d'appui*, a temporary expedient, which a true healer must,
so to speak, inspire with the 'breath of life'. He also avoids
formulas and definitions as far as possible, whereas even
in his medical literature the modern Westerner has a primary interest in specific directives and informative material. These subtleties are very difficult to explain. Essentially it is a matter of profoundly divergent conceptions
of the *raison d'être* of medical literature. According to an
élite rooted in traditional Asian tenets, that which is most
vital is the very thing which cannot be defined. This élite
is doubtful whether it is really possible for the West to
define these crucial issues either. Is it not true, for instance, that the number of Western publications on gerontology and geriatrics over the years totals more than
30,000, but that neither biological nor medical science has
succeeded in defining, even partially, what the ageing
process actually is, or at which point in time it begins?

It is obvious that in the sphere of tradition-oriented
Asian medicine and science, there are also a considerable
number of ignoramuses who avoid definitions because
they are incapable of making reasonable ones. This same
absence of Western clarity and precision encourages op-
portunists to throw the spotlight on pseudo-mystical,
sham wisdom. It is also possible that the so-called secret
domains are used as a facade to cloud the underlying ignorance. There are two sides to everything . . .

The limited number of extant translations and summar-
ies of Lamaist medical texts are a poor reflection of the
originals.[5] For this reason, numerous erroneous opinions

[5] In 1973, however, the first really comprehensive work to appear in
English was published: Rechung, *Tibetan Medicine*, Wellcome. (Tr.)

concerning them are current in the West. Some believe that even the Tibetan medical works considered standard consist mainly of magical formulas and wild speculation. In fact, serious books of this kind often display unmistakable signs of clarity and, one might almost say, scientific precision sometimes almost Western in flavour. This is either apparent immediately, or becomes so upon judicious consideration of the symbolism. Magical formulas and so forth often occupy less than one thousandth part of the contents. They are often only interpolated as a polite gesture towards Lamaism, which rules supreme in the 'Forbidden Land'.[6]

Following this outline of Tibetan medical literature, it might be appropriate to make a few observations about the doctor's status in the 'Forbidden Land', medical training and fees or other forms of remuneration given to serious practitioners of the healing art.

To study Tibetan medicine takes a very long time and is considered particularly arduous. Thirteen years of foundation studies are the usual requirement before starting any medical course as such. The entrance requirements for a medical college involve difficult qualifying examinations. Instruction is both theoretical and practical and many examinations are held at the patient's bedside, where the candidate must treat him under his teacher's supervision. The prestige of the medical profession is so great, that it is not even necessary to give a diploma to a doctor who has been properly examined at a medical college. It is an accepted fact that absolutely no non-doctor would dare to pose as a physician. Quacks are not discouraged. Perhaps they consider that the results of the latter's treatments help to persuade people of the superiority of authentic

[6] Until 1959. (Tr.)

doctors. And if a so-called quack is a really outstanding healer, then some way of integrating him into the medical profession can indeed be found. The title of fully qualified doctor is *men-ram-pa*. Scientific co-operation takes place especially by periodically changing diaries, in which remarks are entered concerning the diagnosis and treatment of particularly instructive, unusual cases of disease.

Until very recently, no genuine central Asian healer requested any fee at all. At the same time, however, healing which goes unrewarded is frowned upon, primarily because in the long run it 'brings no luck' to the person under treatment.

The patient is therefore careful to remunerate the doctor according to his means; usually in the form of natural produce or objects and presents. The voluntary donations of people who are reasonably prosperous are quite considerable, and those of very poor people often extremely meagre. The spiritual effects of each remuneration depend on its relation to the patient's income. The principle applied here is reminiscent of the Bible story about the poor widow's mite. A few years ago I heard from South America, that one of the richest people on the South American continent paid a doctor a fee of millions in the local currency for his cure. Nevertheless, it only amounted to about one five-hundredth of his vast wealth. A true Asian would have considered this patient an outright miser, despite the huge amount he paid! He feels that for a life-saving intervention, it is proper to present a doctor with something which equals a really hard-felt financial loss to the patient. A very poor man, whoever he may be, who repays his doctor's treatment with an exceptionally meagre present which would hardly pay for a couple of cheap meals, is considered very generous by comparison!

At all events, there, where things are less compartmental-ised and valued more from the human point of view, the Asian equivalent of Robert Owen's poem very rarely ap-plies: 'God and the doctor we alike adore – But only when in danger, not before – The danger over, both are alike requited – God is forgotten and the doctor slighted!'

Unscrupulous money-makers in the 'Forbidden Land', who somehow manage to worm their way in amongst genuine healers, have the chance to be much more of a nuisance there than their counterparts in the West. This is partly because the Tibetan healer is also the patient's pharmacist, and can 'feed' him with expensive medicines as it suits him. And if such people happen to succeed in encroaching upon the borders of certain secret teachings, the devastating effect on the environment, and on them-selves too, is so horrifying that it is understandable why an Asian élite should take certain precautionary meas-ures. Not only during the earlier stages of Western devel-opment, but also today, amongst the members of this élite, stress is laid upon the absolute necessity of observing the golden rule of occult science: 'When you attempt to take one step towards knowing hidden truths, you have to take three steps simultaneously towards knowing your own weaknesses and towards the perfection of your char-acter!'

Materia Medica

SINCE Tibetan doctors prefer 'whole person therapies', it is not surprising that their choice of medicines is made primarily in relation to how they affect the whole organism. At the same time, due consideration is also given to local treatment.

The majority of medical substances used are of vegetable origin, the minority animal, and an even smaller proportion mineral.

When gathering medicinal plants, the soil in which they grow must be closely examined. Attention is paid to its quality and condition, whether insects live there or not, and so on. If one is seeking plants to be used in the preparation of medicines for febrile diseases, they must be picked from the northern slopes of the mountains, never from the south. Some drugs must be stored for at least twenty-four hours in an iron container, even when it cannot be proved whether the iron has the slightest effect on the substances in question. Under these circumstances, it is understandable that the compounding of materia medica based on analysis, which is considered extremely important in the West, appears insufficient to the central Asian healing practitioner. This is because the more subtle factors, upon which their effects most often depend, are not taken into account. Thick sugar syrup, for instance, is often used in the preparation of medicinal compounds, but close attention is paid to the subtle difference between syrup which has condensed in the sun and that which has condensed in the shade.

Tibetan pharmacology has access to a wealth of experience accumulated over many centuries. In the large libraries of the 'Forbidden Land', innumerable voluminous works are to be found which deal with the origin, composition, and effects of many curative substances. Not one of them has yet been translated into a Western language.[1]

Reliable, comprehensive works on Tibetan pharmacology are: the *men-dyi-nam-ye-ngo-wo-nu-ming-dye-par-she-pa-dri-me-she-treng* and the *du-shom-pe-nyem-po-tsi-men-dyi-nu-pa-kyang-she-sel-don* (this rendering follows the pronunciation of educated Tibetans). The second title, which begins with the words 'The Conquest of Devils', is just decorative – as often happens in Tibetan literature – and therefore misleading.

These two works deal with the nature and action of many hundreds of medicinal substances derived from the animal, vegetable and mineral kingdoms. Frequently-used remedies are discussed in great detail, sometimes even including information about the taste and the *nu-pa* (roughly : taste action in the patient's stomach).

The second of these volumes deals extensively with, amongst other things, the effect of milk, yoghurt and so forth, which are in a certain sense also considered as aids to healing.

Descriptions are nearly always very lucid and to the point. A text sample : *myristica fragrans* (nutmeg) cor-

---

[1] Except the chapters from the *bshad-rgyud* in *Tibetan Medicine* by Rechung, 1973. (Tr.)

rects the prevalence of air. *Chu-gang* (gypsum taken internally) helps in feverish affections, particularly of the lungs, and dispels traumatic fever.

The identification of materia medica is not always easy, even for Tibetan pharmacologists, since slight name changes used to occur frequently from one province to another within Tibet. In China too, where they are falling back increasingly nowadays on the store of ancient Chinese medical experience, the attempt to establish consistent norms in pharmacology is encountering great difficulties. The same medicinal plant is often designated quite differently, even by specialists, in different parts of China.

The same applies to the healing art in other Asian countries. An account of various ancient Indian pharmacological preparations, sent to me from India in December 1956, contained the following significant observation : "In some cases it is now no longer possible, even for the most erudite physicians, well versed in the principles of the ancient Indian healing art, and with the best will in the world, to ascertain which modern drugs correspond to the substances prescribed in their time-honoured treatises!"

Amongst the substances derived from the animal kingdom, they use powdered bone-segments (sometimes antlers), the flesh, blood, bile, fat, brains, skin and so forth of various animals. Amongst other things, they attribute a powerful healing action to a substance which forms in the gall-bladder of diseased horned cattle. From the parts of plants, they use roots, stems, trunks, branches, bark, rind, leaves, blossoms and fruit.

Medicaments are administered in the form of embrocations, medicinal baths, enemas, inhalations, fumigations and burning incense. For oral ingestion : decoctions, lixiviations, extracts obtained by crushing, and powders of curative substances made up into pills or capsules. The purpose of this is not so much to spare the patient the unpleasant taste of certain medicines as to produce a particular curative effect.

There are no fixed rules at all concerning the duration of medical treatments. They sometimes have to be continued for a whole year, in which case, of course, suitable intermissions and variations are incorporated in order to prevent the patient becoming habituated to medicaments administered over such a long period. Cases are even known in which medicines had to be taken for a total of three years. Both in the treatment of leprosy – which the Tibetan, like the Indian doctor, divides into eighteen categories – and of senility, medicines are dispensed over particularly long periods. In general, however, medicinal treatments are restricted to shorter periods.

The number of remedies used in Tibetan medicine is very large. Theoretically it is probably greater than the number of medicaments which traditional Chinese medicine employs. The *Pen Tsao Kang Mu*, one of the most important Chinese works on pharmacology by the famous sixteenth century Chinese pharmacologist Li Shih-chen, enumerates roughly two thousand different substances. In practice, however, this vast selection diminishes. The remedies most frequently used in Tibetan medicine too, only amount to a fraction of the quantity mentioned above.

The number of prescriptions in Tibet is purported to be even greater than the ten thousand Chinese written up in the *Pen Tsao Kang Mu*.

Amongst the many healing substances which play a part in Lamaist pharmacology, let us mention the following:

MATERIA MEDICA	USES
Aesculus sinensis (a variety of horse-chestnut)	The preparation of strong emetics.
Cuscuta sinensis (clover dodder)	To counteract hot diseases of the lungs, liver and blood vessels.
Artemisia capillaris (mugwort)	For hot lung complaints.
Gardenia florida	For hot diseases of the gall-bladder and liver.
Hemp	Diseases of the lymphatic vessels; skin complaints.
Finely powdered iron	For afflictions of the lungs; to neutralize poisons in the liver; for eye complaints.
Finely powdered gold	For diseases of the heart, liver, gall-bladder, lungs and joints. .
Verdigris (great caution as to dosage!)	To counteract a series of hot diseases; to assuage pain.
Gypsum (for internal use)	To lower the overall temperature; in Tibetan medicine particularly for lung diseases and for traumatic fever; in traditional Chinese medicine for many serious febrile conditions, including epidemic encephalitis.
Calcite (finely powdered)	To strengthen the bones; taken internally to accelerate the mending of broken bones; in hot phlegm diseases.

Ginseng	To neutralize poisons in the body; to rejuvenate ageing people.
Foeniculum vulgare (fennel)	For most hot air diseases; as a detoxicating agent; for eye complaints.
Malachite	For hot bone diseases; for treating the eyes; to restrict the flow of lymph.
Nepeta japonica (catmint or catnip)	In the preparation of anodynes.
Indigo	For treating the eyes; for burns.
Liquorice	To counteract loss of weight; for lung diseases; to assuage pain.
Strychnos nux-vomica (vomit nut)	For hot stomach diseases. (Warning against overdoses in view of mental disturbances.)
Musk	In shaking fits; cancer; diseases of the ears; kidney diseases; febrile states brought about by mental factors.
Senecia sagittatus (a groundsel)	For healing wounds; for eye infections.

In identifying Tibetan materia medica one can easily slip up and make serious mistakes. For example: *ne-zen* is a substance sometimes used for healing purposes. In a Western translation it was rendered as 'sparrow's flesh'. What it really means though is barley-corn which has been eaten by sparrows and partly processed in the digestive tract, then removed from the entrails of recently dead sparrows and used as an admixture in medicinal compounds. Obviously the person who witnessed the procedure did not pay close attention.

In addition to the actual language difficulties, the understanding of Tibetan pharmacology is sometimes aggravated by a tendency to make medical compilations from totally foreign frames of reference. One such grouping divides materia medica according to 'spheres'; a particular substance is considered typical for each specific sphere, and for this reason especially potent healing properties are attributed to it. According to the *gyu-shi*, the following belong to these 'typical' and therefore especially effective remedies:

1. *Drag-shun* (mineral pitch, bitumen), a viscous substance which forms on rock. It is rich in 'earth elements' and is supposed to be a particularly effective ingredient in medicinal compounds for diseases of the musculature.[2]

2. *Chong-shi* (calcite) is described as especially rich in 'stone energy'.

3. Treacle embodies the 'essence' of the trees and is considered 'typical' in the sphere of tonics.

4. Honey is considered the 'essence of the flower kingdom'. It reinforces *dang*, a Tibetan word which can only be translated very roughly as 'vital glow', like that visible in the natural facial colouring, sparkling eyes and so forth, of healthy people.

5. Fresh butter, which abounds in the essence of grass and is also particularly rich in *chu*, an expression which roughly corresponds to 'concentrated vitality'.

Mineral pitch (bitumen) is also considered a particularly effective remedy for lowering the temperature and is em-

---

[2] i.e., 'typical' in the sphere of such diseases. (Tr.)

ployed as an admixture in medicines for many organic afflictions (stomach, liver etc.). Calcite is said to encourage the mending of bones, whilst treacle and honey are amongst those substances most frequently used for 'binding' medicines, as well as being employed internally and as an embrocation. Honey is also applied, usually in combination with oil, in the after-care of areas which have suffered as a result of energetic fire therapies undertaken for curative purposes.

The substance in which a medicine is dispensed, which in other words 'carries' the medicine, is called *men-ta* or 'medicine horse'. Apart from water and alcohol (usually in the form of strong, hot Tibetan beer), the most frequent 'medicine horses' are sugar, treacle and honey. The effects of many medicinal ingredients are also supposed to vary according to whether they are dispensed in sugar, let us say, or in treacle.

A practical general rule, which nearly every Tibetan healer (who is at the same time also an apothecary) knows by heart, runs as follows:

ka-ra-thrag-thri-tsa-wa-sel-we-ta
men-ta-bu-ram-drang-lung-sel-we-ta
drang-tsi-be-ken-chu-ser-sel-we-ta

This means:

'Sugar is a (very appropriate) medicine horse for dispelling hot blood and (hot) bile; treacle as a medicine horse is suitable for curing cold air diseases;
honey is the appropriate medicine horse for overcoming phlegm and (excessive) lymph.'

Tibetan doctors occasionally coat their medicinal compounds with resinous substances, so that they pass unaffected through the stomach, and do not take effect until they reach that part of the intestine intended by the healer.

Many dietary specifications belong to the fringe areas of Tibetan pharmacology. Since a good many of these are based on centuries of experience, they are well worth looking into. It should be remembered, however, that the central Asian sometimes reacts differently from the Westerner, even under the same external conditions. In the interests of maintaining health, certain foods should not constitute part of the same meal: for example fish and milk, honey and melted butter, milk and fruit or flesh of fowl and yoghurt. Tibetan diatetics and pharmaceutics go more by the conviction of the relative value of food and drink than their Western counterparts do.

Classical Chinese medicine also speaks sometimes of 'dangerous combinations of foodstuffs', like hens' eggs and garlic or onions, which is said to create a tendency to shortness of breath.

Whereas Tibetan pharmacology and its fringe areas cover a wide range of factors which Western science does not heed, it has on the other hand little appreciation of the painstaking precision which is the tool of the Western pharmacologist. It does not reckon in grammes and milligrammes, but to 'pea-size' and a 'quantity corresponding to an Indian sesame seed' – which is very tiny – and so on. Exactitude is probably avoided on purpose, in the same way as the entire medical nomenclature – in spite of the enormous vocabulary of the Tibetan language and the nuances of which it is capable – is intentionally unspecific about many things. This is probably partly to discourage newcomers to the profession from relying too heavily on definitions and 'tools'.

So-called 'sewage pharmacy' is less abundant in Tibetan than in classical Chinese medicine. This type of pharmacy makes use of the excrement and urine of various living creatures; for example imported elephant urine is used to supplement medicines for the treatment of intestinal worms. But contrary to ancient Chinese 'sewage pharmacology', there is hardly ever any mention in the Tibetan of such 'horrifying substances' as poisonous fungi growing on corpses in buried coffins, or tooth-tartar, ear-wax, urine sediments, sweat, dandruff, and so on. Those who feel inclined to ridicule these things might consider the fact that, with penicillin and similar achievements of recent years, we too have moved into a field which is basically not so very far removed from these 'unappetising' substances.

On the basis of comparisons between different Tibetan medical texts, I have endeavoured to establish what effects the most commonly used healing substances exert upon the humours. It should be remembered that air diseases occur most frequently in Tibet. One computation yields that there are one hundred and ten remedies which inhibit all three humours to varying degrees. Ninety-two substances serve to eliminate the excess of air, thirty do the same for bile, forty for phlegm disturbances, and forty-six remedies help to treat two humours simultaneously. Examples of remedies which inhibit air are santal (sandalwood), betel and camphor. Agents used for treating a prevalence of bile are *zizyphus vulgaris* (common jujube), *polyganatum multiflorum* (many flowered Solomon's seal) and *campanula trachelium* (throatwort or blue foxglove). Agents for reducing phlegm are *ligustrum lucidum* (yellow privet), *momordica monadelpha* (a variety of cucumber) and *cydonia sinensis* (quince).

Some of the remedies valued for lowering high temperatures are ginseng, *carthanus tinctorius* (safflower), cinnabar, *cuscuta sinensis* (variety of dodder) and *artemisia capillaris* (mugwort, a species of the wormwood genus);

for raising the temperature: *aconitum fischeri* (a variety of monkshood), *piper nigrum* (black pepper) and *vitex trifoliata*. Experience shows that healing substances which lower the temperature are in the majority.

A very important consideration for the Tibetan healer is whether the effect of a curative agent used to inhibit the over-production of a certain humour, leaves the rest un-affected, or whether it creates a predisposition towards an abnormal ebullition of the other humours. The Lamaist doctor has access to medical reference books for details on this, all of which he cannot, of course, keep in his head. Most remedies with a 'burning' taste, for instance, includ-ing the respective spices, have a tendency to diminish air as well as phlegm. But it is explicitly stated in pharmaco-logical texts, that they simultaneously produce an ebulli-tion of bile if the particular medicinal compound used does not contain the addition of *piper longum* and/or gin-ger. It is repeatedly stressed that such an ebullition of an-other humour only occurs when the medicines adminis-tered to inhibit the first humour or humours are dispensed in excess. In characteristic Tibetan fashion, they do not find it necessary to give any information on exact propor-tions, or what in fact is to be understood by an overdose. This is left to the personal discretion of the healer, since these things have to be individually adjusted to each parti-cular case.

All in all, Tibetan pharmacological literature is hardly any less copious than that of the West today. An exhaust-ive description covering even only a part of the wide field of Tibetan pharmacology would comprise an entire series of thick volumes. In this book, therefore, I can only pick out a few details, which should serve to promote a better understanding of Tibetan medicine in its totality.

Let us examine a few examples of the group of medications used for treating individual organs.

Heart Diseases

A beneficial action upon heart ailments is attributed to the following remedies in particular: powdered gold, the *nying-sho-sha* (a sister plant of *canavalia gladiata*, related to the bean genus) and, especially for heart complaints caused by an excess of air, nutmeg and *asa foetida*. In such cases, moreover, the use of aconite is recommended (with caution, of course, because of its poisonous properties), and also calamus, musk and frankincense – taken internally in this case. In heart complaints accompanied by pain, the principal recommendation is a decoction of a mixture of nutmeg, fennel and the above-mentioned *nying-sho-sha*, with a dash of powdered costus-root and *caryophyllus aromaticus* (clove). For hot heart afflictions the Tibetan doctor advises a sugar-based mixture of camphor, *nying-sho-sha*, nutmeg, bear's bile and the Tibetan *chu-gang*, which is almost the equivalent of gypsum in the West. The latter is also frequently used in traditional Chinese medicine, and in 1955 is reported to have produced exceptional results in the fight against *encephalitis lethargica* at a large Chinese children's clinic. It was here that practical co-operation was instigated between Western-style doctors and healing practitioners working along the lines of conventional Asian medicine.

Liver Complaints

Saffron is advised in by far the majority of liver complaints. The use of this remedy is very widespread in Tibetan healing and Chinese medicine has also employed it for centuries. Other substances which Tibeto-Lamaist medicine uses for the treatment of liver affections include iron rust and *gleditschia sinensis*. For cold liver complaints *caryophyllus aromaticus* (clove) and a central Asian species of cumin known as *zi-ra* are used. Medicines recommended for hot liver diseases are cinnabar and pure, powdered copper.

Stomach Diseases

Cinnamon bark is recommended for cold stomach disorders in which an ebullition of air is also involved. Lime is the principal prescription for mucous stomach blockages and stomach ulcers. *Punica granatum* (pomegranate) is reputed to act favourably upon virtually all stomach affections. Remedial successes are attributed to mineral pitch (bitumen), especially in hot disorders of the stomach, liver and kidneys. Coriander is also said to be effective in the treatment of hot mucous formations in the stomach, whilst *caryophyllus aromaticus* acts favourably upon cold stomach complaints which constrict the digestive process.

Eye Diseases

Remedies for counteracting eye disorders characterised by 'congestion', which are precisely the opposite of those indicated by excessive watering: *Valeriana officinalis*, musk, *elettaria cardamomum*, sandalwood, saffron, realgar, and small admixtures of ginger and *piper longum* (with a careful choice of 'medicine horse' to suit the particular ebullition of humours).

In 'lacrimal diseases' caused by a prevalence of air: a mixture of saffron with old butter is boiled in water then introduced into the patient's nostrils.

For 'lacrimal diseases' in excessive bile conditions: lubrication of the eyes with a salve compounded of camphor, human milk and bear's bile in a honey base.

For 'lacrimal diseases' caused by phlegm : lubrication of the eyes with very small quantities of realgar and *piper longum* in a honey base. Post-treatment with a water-based suspension of white sandalwood and liquorice.

In Tibetan texts not regarded primarily as medical books, references are to be found recommending indigo for most eye disorders. They also recommend magnesium containing iron for ocular opacity (probably corneal affections) and *tha-ram* (in reference books, *plantago major vulgaris latifolia, variatio asiatica*) for the relief of corneal affections and redness of the eyes.

For identifying materia medica, it should also be noted that, apart from a really thorough knowledge of the Tibetan language and its many specialised medical and pharmacological terms (of which even the largest dictionaries contain only a few), a good knowledge of the conditions in Tibet is required too. For example, a detailed Tibetan pharmacological work states that soda has a salty taste. Only one familiar with Tibetan conditions would realise straight away that it must mean Tibetan soda, which is procured from the salt lakes of Tibet and therefore does indeed have a salty taste, which masks the basic soda flavour. One must also be prepared for many other difficulties. In a medical discipline, for instance, which utilises quite a number of animal substances, one is inclined to presume that words like 'horseshoe' or 'pig's head' in pharmacological texts, actually refer to specific animal substances. In fact, what are meant here are medicinal plants not found in dictionaries and reference books.

Many medicinal substances used in Tibet and neighbouring countries have to be imported. But even indigenous substances, like bear's bile, certain pulverised semi-precious stones and so forth, are often difficult to obtain and are not cheap. Years ago in China, bear's bile cost more than ten dollars per ounce, whilst powdered rhinoceros horn – used both in Tibetan and Chinese medicine – cost not less than twenty dollars per ounce, even in those days. When converted (the so-called Mexican dollar was worth roughly half an American dollar) this amounts to no less than £177 per kilogram![3]

The ginseng root, known in Tibetan medicine as *kar-po-chig-thub*, the medicinal plant of long life, is also very expensive. It is imported from other parts of East Asia, especially Korea. If ginseng is cultivated in an artificial setting, it behaves just like most creative people persuaded to integrate into the bustle of modern man's gigantic machine-age 'apparatus': it revolts, inasmuch as it simply stops producing active healing substances although continuing to appear to the outside world to be real ginseng. So, it must just be left in the jungle setting, continually tended, whereupon, after six to seven years patient attendance, it begins to accumulate healing powers. Although for most healing purposes less than one hundredth of a gramme of this precious plant is usually ample, treatment is nevertheless so expensive that repeated attempts are made (hitherto in vain) to substitute ginseng by other products.

Ginseng is mainly used to rejuvenate the human body. Entire chapters in Tibetan medical literature are devoted to that branch of knowledge which has recently become more or less commonly known in the West as 'gerontology' and 'geriatrics'. This of course is a sphere in which the Tibetans view momentary successes as least desirable. This is because such successes have to be paid for some months or years later with very unpleasant

[3] This was in 1957. (Tr.)

side-effects, which render the affected person even more senile. Tibetan methods of treatment for the ageing are nearly always of long duration, and a six month course of medicinal treatment is not rare. Results are said to appear only during the course of the next few years. The main substances used are those geared to the overall regeneration of the organism by encouraging the intake of large amounts of chu.[4]

The ageing person who goes to a genuine healer, who is not concerned with making money, is bound to encounter little understanding or encouragement if he wants to draw out his life a little longer solely for the purpose of enjoyment. The creative person, on the other hand, who is growing older and conceives of his earthly existence as a mission, will usually find him a source of real support and unfailing help. Generally speaking, in serious Tibetan medical works, a man who would lengthen his life is advised, apart from a régime of special treatments and long-term courses of medicines, to live where possible in clean housing conditions (not only material), and, whenever possible, to stay by himself in places free from noise, which are also harmonious with respect to plants and animals.

[4] Page 48.

Tibetan Methods of Healing

AS A RESULT of the doctrine of the three humours in Tibetan medicine, the methods of treatment which act on the disordered humours are very extensive. Cases of disease in which one particular humour has gone completely overboard in all areas and 'on every level' are relatively rare. This type poses the least problems. The situation is much more complicated when it involves primary and secondary, or subtle and gross humoral disharmonies (in the sense we discussed earlier); when the illness is attributable to the ebullition of several humours; or when the imbalance of one or more humours is limited to particular levels of the patient's being. The higher the levels of being concerned, the more they belong to the spiritual sphere and the more complex the healing methods and medicinal compounds usually become. Thus it can happen that in an oral disease – Tibetan cosmology accords the highest level of being to the mouth – a medical preparation might contain thirty to forty different ingredients, and making up the prescription could take the doctor an entire day of painstaking effort. This is because on this highest of levels, nearly every influence can be either harmful or beneficial, and the doctor must work carefully through a labyrinth of compromises. From such cases, however, let us return to the simplest: those which involve an overall prevalence of one of the three humours.

The healer will direct his attention to include spiritual factors, even in the treatment of the simplest cases. In most instances of air diseases, this will involve removing the patient's 'spiritual pride', along with giving medicinal treatment; or in phlegm illnesses, working on his ignorance in spiritual matters. It is important to ensure that such influences have a correct correspondence: that the whole psychological make-up of the sick person is kept in mind. Hence it makes a great difference whether a person is of no special significance in spiritual matters, feels himself superior to others, or whether a really creative person is aware of his own worth. Even 'spiritual wrath' can be justified in some cases, whereas an egotistical, wild rage is indicative of a person who acts out his life similarly in other respects. It is appropriate likewise, to see everything not just in a mechanical routine way, but rather from a spiritual viewpoint. This of course applies to the tendency in Tibetan medicine as a whole to take additional consideration of those factors which in the West are generally regarded as the domain of the priest or psychiatrist.

The Tibetan physician divides his practical methods into the following categories:

1. *che*. (In this book I use the phonetic rendering of Tibetan terms which comes closest to the pronunciation of the *Lha-sa* dialect – a sort of lingua franca in Tibet.)

Belonging to *che* are:

(a) the *jam-pe-che* or gentle methods: burning incense (the Tibetan work *kun-dzob-ya-sel-me-long* lists twelve different types of incense); the use of herbal mixtures, various animal substances and chemicals, medicinal baths, rubbing salves into the skin, the nostrils, etc.

(b) the *tsub-che* or stronger methods: bloodletting, vigorous Tibetan treatments, the lancing of abcesses, etc.

(c) the *drag-po-che* or violent, radical methods: surgical operations (which, although practised far more rarely than in the West, are not unknown in Tibet), the painful removal of foreign bodies, cauterization of abcesses, curetting of severely damaged tissues, etc.

It should be noted here, that the Tibetan, like other Asians, can endure even major operations without anaesthetics because he is far less sensitive to pain than the average Westerner. The enormous progress during the last few decades in the sphere of pain-relief makes the Westerner much less capable of enduring pain.

It should also be mentioned that in some cases, in which he could very easily relieve pain, the Tibetan doctor deems it undesirable to do so, as for example in the treatment of venereal diseases. This is due to considerations which reveal a strict moral code.

2. The prescription of a diet adapted to the disease.

3. *Jong*, which can be roughly translated as cleansing. This method primarily involves emetics and laxatives.

4. The administration of medicines, which are the subject of a separate chapter in this book.

Let us begin with the simplest diseases: those directly caused by a general excess of one of the three humours on all levels. In bile diseases of this type, Tibetan medical texts primarily recommend radical purgatives, bloodletting and rubbing the body with cold water.

For diseases characterised in general by air, a beneficial effect is best obtained from embrocations of old butter, combined with massage, especially around the crown of the patient's head, if done with great care. It must be added that not only the taste, but also the odour of butter, however old, is agreeable to Tibetans. As a special treat at Tibetan celebration feasts, dishes are sometimes served which are prepared with butter which is several years old! Many Lamaist doctors also stock a certain amount of butter which is at least one year old amongst their supplies. There are two main types of massage in Tibet, which are performed not only manually but sometimes also with heated stones. Burning incense and fumigations prepared with medicaments high in fat content are also suitable for combating air diseases; also the administration of mild purgatives and a number of heat and sweat treatments.

In phlegm diseases the Tibetan doctor usually prescribes an emetic treatment immediately, later combined with a series of the above-mentioned *drag-po-che* (such as vigorous fire treatments and so on). Milder interventions, such as physical exercises, are also an integral part of combating phlegm. Massages with butter are also given to reduce excess phlegm; here fresh butter is usually preferred.

The administration of sternutatories is applicable in both phlegm and air diseases. Bloodletting is particularly appropriate in the case of bile affections which have encroached upon the blood system, although this does not always mean 'blood' in the customary Western sense.

Many Tibetan curative methods only correspond superficially to Western ones, although they seem to serve similar ends. Extreme caution is advised concerning emetic and purgative treatments, for instance. A good Tibetan doctor should never administer laxatives – of which Tibetan pharmacology describes at least one hundred and thirty-three varieties – without first preparing the patient. The same applies to emetics. The *gyu-shi* states that a healer who dispenses purgatives or emetics without preparatory treatment is acting like a fool 'who

pours cold water on ice to thaw it out'. In the Tibetan
view, which perhaps includes certain subtle aspects here,
this kind of practice tends to putrefy the organism even
more. Preparation of the patient consists partly of administering loosening agents. These include *piper longum*
and cinammon bark for emetic treatments. In illnesses
characterised distinctively by phlegm, the admixture of
fresh butter is recommended as an emetic or loosening
agent.

One of the features of Tibetan preventative medicine
which seems odd to the Western doctor is the repeatedly
stressed warning against sleeping during the daytime. It
can apparently have unpleasant effects on one's health.
There are exceptions, of course, such as certain cases of
mental illness, or people with a disposition towards air
who require sleep on hot summer afternoons to gain
strength. Nevertheless, even in exceptional cases, sleep
during the day is carefully rationed by the doctor. Indeed, it is often only permitted as a 'medicine' when the
number of breaths drawn during sleep are carefully
counted. In cases of disease where Tibetans consider sleep
during the day to be particularly harmful, the patient's
relatives are strongly urged to watch over the sick-bed
in the daytime to see that he does not fall asleep, and to
rouse him immediately if he dozes off. It is especially
inadvisable for people who are predisposed to phlegm
affections to sleep during the day. In such cases Tibetans
believe that the latter, particularly, can 'drag along' the
remaining humours; in other words, it can lead to a com-
plication in the phlegm disease by disturbing the other
two humours.

Likewise, sexual intercourse during the daytime should
be avoided by people who have a tendency to suffer from

ulcers. Generally speaking, sexual intercourse is considered harmful in the early morning and during the evening.

Other healing practices rarely employed in the West are: hitting and applying pressure to individual joints and a treatment which subjects the patient to a series of contrasts, by alternately clothing and unclothing him completely. Fasting is only advised in very rare cases. Generally speaking, loss of appetite and digestive disorders are regarded as much more serious symptoms than in the West. Tibetan medicine firmly believes that disturbed assimilation and digestion are a sign of very grave dangers. It therefore pays a great deal of attention to restoring regular function of the stomach, intestine, and lymphatic system. Lymph is called 'yellow water' in Tibetan medicine. The *gyu-shi*, one of the foremost Lamaist medical works, points emphatically to the pathological excess of lymph as the precipitating cause of a host of the most serious diseases, including leprosy. According to scholarly opinion in central Asia, the actual infection is nearly always just the final outcome of a whole series of more deep-rooted causes, which gradually 'ripen' the afflicted person for the disease. The severest forms of dropsy are also included in this category, whilst tuberculosis is held to be due to precisely the opposite: insufficient lymph production.

In very simple digestive complaints, which are not linked with any organic causes whatever, Tibetan doctors prescribe taking frequent small quantities of hot water, followed each time by a massage of the stomach area with the palm of the hand.

It has already been mentioned that many therapies and medicines can serve to treat disturbances involving not just one, but sometimes two, and more rarely, all three humours. The greater the skill and knowledge of the doctor, the more he is in a position to select those procedures from amongst the numerous ones available to him. By intentionally limiting their effect, he can channel them in a specific direction, in order to overcome perhaps only one particular aspect of the evil. Doing so depends more on the doctor's initiative and his ability to assess the situation than on any hard and fast rules. This is because the same remedy can effect two different humours, depending on whether it is dispensed in a concentrated form, perhaps as powder, or as an infusion in the form of tea.

Acupuncture, in spite of its recognised success, is generally only practised with care and reserve. This is probably due to the postulation that the essence of this method, which is deemed to have more than just passing effects, is so difficult to learn that it necessitates training of a demanding nature lasting several decades, and including whenever possible certain occult studies as well. In other words, it should only be practised by very highly qualified specialists.

Acupuncture, as is well known, has been practised for centuries in Chinese medicine. It is purported to be sometimes successful where the rest of medical science fails. According to a Chinese doctor – who, by virtue of his championship of acupuncture, has also made a name for himself in Europe – acupuncture is but little understood even in China. In saying this, however, he was most probably referring to the spiritual foundations. In fact, the knowledge embodied in these foundations has the status of an esoteric science in China. Acupuncture is often only applied on a purely technical basis today, even by traditional healers. The mechanics of this system – the choice of needles, disinfecting them and the technique of insertion – can be conveyed to any marginally intelligent person within half an hour. Even the different points of insertion – now nearly nine hundred – can be learned within months. In traditional Chinese medical schools, models of the naked human body, showing all the points, are constructed in bronze for this purpose. They are freshly covered with wax before every lesson, so that the student can conveniently ascertain in a practical way whether or not his needle has pierced the prescribed point. Over the centuries, even traditional Chinese healers have increasingly pushed the mechanical side of acupuncture into the foreground. It is not easy to discover what this healing method really involves, nor even some of its hidden dangers. This is because, according to the Asian physician, currents of life force, invisible and eluding material qualification, circulate throughout the human body. Any skilled intervention must take the rhythm of these currents into account. In the opinion of Asian scholars on a particularly high level, many modern acupuncturists are wrong when they reject as superstition the observation of forbidden seasons, days and hours for the insertion of needles.

Moxa or moxibustion goes hand in hand with acupuncture. It consists of burning an aromatic species of plant, similar to mugwort and called *ai* in Chinese, over the surface of the skin at particular, precisely designated points. The fact that the same plant species is also used in exorcism indicates that the subtle level plays a part here too. Be that as it may, moxa certainly has a favourable influence on the course of disease in many cases. Doctors of the Western school outside Tibet and China have established unequivocally that it leads to a surprisingly large increase in blood corpuscles, both red and white.

Practices similar to moxa, in contrast to acupuncture, are quite frequent in Tibetan medicine, which recognises, in addition, a whole series of other heat treatments which would take too much space to describe here in detail. They range from almost painless procedures similar to moxa to practices which appear excessively cruel to modern Westerners. An example of the latter is the treatment of diseased joints and bones by pouring boiling oil into incisions, which should not be too far from the diseased spot, and not too close either, to avoid any serious damage by excessive heat to the part of the body under treatment. It is obvious that, particularly in such instances, the ability of central Asians to withstand a great deal more pain and the consequences of radical interventions is an integral factor. Such methods cannot be just imitated elsewhere.

Tibetan and ancient Indian medicine distinguish, all in all, between at least thirteen different healing methods connected with special heat treatments and sweat-cures using heated brass rods, steam, hot stones, heated sand-packs and so on. Heat cures which would directly affect the eyes or sexual organs are always avoided when possible. For surface operations the actual burning and singeing is performed with open metal containers in which a quantity of combustible material is lit, and then placed on the patient's skin. In major operations, such as the radical cauterization of malignant tumours, there are instruments, which, in spite of their primitiveness, are quite similar to some Western ones. They differ, however, in that their shape sometimes reveals adaptations to the so-called 'magic cosmology',[1] inasmuch as they are reminiscent of

[1] c.f. Rechung, *Tibetan Medicine*, pp. 82-84. (Tr.)

animal figures which either exist on the physical level, or allegedly belong to the 'intermediate world' between matter and pure spirit.

There is a widespread opinion, even amongst people who have to some extent come to grips with questions about central Asian medicine, that the traditional Asian healing art, especially in China and Tibet, refrains, virtually without exception, from performing any surgical operations whatever. This view does not tally with the facts. As early as the second century A.D. the famous doctor Hua-to, for example, performed stomach operations after anaesthetizing the patient with a 'dream medicine' (certain drugs). He sometimes even removed severely diseased sections of the intestines, sewed the remaining healthy parts together again and then spread a whitish powder over the wounds to prevent infection. This probably had an effect similar to penicillin.

Tibetan doctors sometimes also perform surgical operations. However, they will only employ their operation techniques, which are incomparably more primitive than ours, when it is absolutely necessary and there is no possible alternative. This is not only because they are aware of the shortcomings of their surgery, but also because of their particular medical philosophy.

To this must be added their radical rejection of blood transfusions, which have of course become a significant part of our modern surgical techniques. Central Asian sages are in accord with the words of the poet, since for them too blood is 'a very special fluid'. It has not only material aspects but also mental-spiritual ones. If, for instance, someone receives blood from a donor who has a tendency to be dishonest, then this transfusion 'infects' the recipient on subtle levels and can encourage the development of any existing dishonest traits. Large scale blood transfusions performed solely from a physical viewpoint, strike the most radical central Asian élitist minds as being, beyond question, 'interventions into spiritual domains perpetrated in folly'. The splendid results of this practice are dearly bought – at the cost of less easily perceptible repercussions on other levels. It is no wonder then that the central Asian healer does not care much for injections, which the modern educated Tibetan refers to as *khab-len*.

The Lamaist doctor's various surgical and other instruments are precisely described in the chapters devoted to *cha-je*, working tools, in different Lamaist medical works. Descriptions include information concerning their measurements in *sor*, which means roughly finger width. I drew the following examples from various long lists: lancets for opening abscesses; saws and drilling devices for bone manipulation; small forceps and similar instruments for removing nodular neoplasms in the throat, nose and auditory canal; an instrument for use in miscarriages; appliances shaped like the head of a snake for removing foreign bodies; contrivances for the radical fire treatment of malignant tumours; a type of lancet called *tsag-bu* for use in bloodletting; small tweezers for removing hair called a *mang-ster*, and so on.

For taking larger amounts of blood, the Tibetan healer employs the *ngab-ru*. It is a horn-shaped instrument which is applied after making an incision with the above-mentioned *tsag-bu*. The healer then begins to suck on the other end until the required amount of blood is obtained.

Then there are devices for blowing medicaments into the nostrils, apparatus for inhaling, and small, curved metal bars for cauterizing the roots of teeth. As far as dentistry is concerned, Tibetan medicine regards dental troubles primarily as an expression of general disharmony, sometimes on very subtle levels. Such troubles affect the whole organism. Traditional Chinese medicine also seems to have taken a similar standpoint, because throughout that vast country, well into the twentieth century, there were only four hundred dentists; in other words less than one for every million inhabitants!

Because his surgical instruments are relatively crude, the Tibetan healer has often been forced to invent alternative methods. There is, for instance, a very simple procedure in Tibet for removing needles, nails and other small iron objects which have been swallowed and could perforate the digestive organs. After flushing the patient's stomach with a fluid intake tempered with suitable medicaments, cotton which has been thoroughly reduced to fibres is administered, together with a large quantity of water and small lumps of magnetised iron ore. The patient is then laid on his stomach and vomits, so that often the entire stomach content is expelled, together with the foreign body which has been attracted by the magnetised iron ore. In this way the patient is put to rights without an operation or any complex interventions. The addition of cotton is important since it helps to envelop the foreign body and prevents damage to the oesophagus.

In the course of my studies of Tibetan ophthalmology (in the *men-ngag-dyu-kyi-len-tab*, the *gyu-shi*, and various ophthalmological references in the *pe-ma-ling-pe-ter-ma*, the *yon-ten-tse-me-pe-ter-ma* etc.) I also came across a reference to a primitive surgical operation practised in this field. In the case of a disease called *ling-thog*, in which the eyes become cloudy and turbid (it will only be possible to ascertain the precise Western equivalent in the event of clinical co-operation between Western ophthalmologists and Tibetan healers), the healer ventures to scale the patient's diseased eye or eyes with a small iron hook, after smearing the eyes with a mixture of malachite, camphor, musk, finely powdered gypsum, saffron and sugar, bathing them with moist medicaments and fumigating them with the steam of heated sealing wax.

Minor surgical operations include tenotomy – especially of the fourth finger – which can have overall repercussions that seem disproportionately far-reaching. This is a general rule which also applies to certain local operations on the hand, and to the action of fire. Under certain circumstances, for instance, mild scorching of all ten fingers is supposed to overcome weak conditions, and a vigorous fire treatment of the ball of the hand to relieve head and toothaches. A Western commentator of a sarcastic disposition said to me in response to this that it could easily be explained, since with such rough treatment the patient's hand must hurt so much that he forgets his head or toothache!

Bloodletting is performed at a wide variety of points. When drawing blood, the healer not only has to select the right points for the particular case, but he must also take the circulation of the life force into account (see page 25). The Tibetan healer recognises seventy-seven bloodletting points. The one to be used is determined primarily by the organs suffering from disease, though it is not always in their immediate location. The tip of the nose and the frontal vein, for example, are the bloodletting points prescribed for eye diseases characterized by 'moist accumulations', of which there are thirty-three. These diseases are associated with ocular congestion and are probably the exact opposite of those associated with excessive watering of the eyes.

In many cases where the Western doctor would step in

immediately, the central Asian healer will simply let nature take its course, despite the multiplicity of his healing methods. For instance, he will only take action to combat nose-bleeding if the loss of blood increases to the point of becoming a real threat to life. Nosebleeding is generally considered a useful prophylactic reaction of the body and should, especially in cancer and many illnesses seated in the head, only be stopped in exceptional cases.

Dermatology is quite a large branch of Tibetan medicine. Skin diseases were very widespread in the 'Forbidden Land' until just recently. This was, of course, partly due to the – by Western standards – hair-raising filth common amongst many ordinary Tibetans. Whereas it was possible, not long ago, to encounter people in remote parts of Eastern Europe, who bathed themselves a few times a year at most, in Tibet there were quite a number who virtually never had a proper wash. Many of the Tibetan people's ablutions were more of a religious or symbolic nature than for purposes of personal hygiene. Only the upper stratum of society were an exception. During the period between the two World Wars, I had the opportunity to observe how higher ranking Tibetans on their travels carried portable baths with them, often in full view.

The fact that widespread uncleanliness amongst ordinary Tibetans did not lead more frequently to epidemics is primarily attributable to the extremely dry alpine climate, which is unfavourable to the development of germs. Regarding the 'neglect' of personal hygiene, however, other factors have to be considered. A Tibetan once told me: 'Pure thoughts are incomparably more important than bodily cleanliness!' It is possible, moreover, that the reason many Tibetans, even the more sophisticated ones, are so water-shy, is because water is said to tend to collect vital energy. This can lead to devitalization of the organism if the surface of the body comes into contact with water too often. Even very tolerant healers also believe that bodily contact with water should be reduced to a minimum, especially in phlegm diseases, whilst in bile diseases washing with hot water particularly should be avoided.

The cause of many skin diseases is considered to lie in the fact that phlegm and/or bile are pulled along by air ebullitions, which then result in phlegm deposits under the surface of the skin. In most cases, however, they are considered symptoms of more far-reaching health disturbances. Tibetan healers deem 'any fool, having once experimented around at length with poisons and plant extracts, capable of making rashes and so forth disappear quickly by concocting mixtures'. But to be able to recognise the disease as a symptom of a much more deep-seated malady, and to cure it at its roots 'is the business of a real physician'. It is said that skin diseases are often the result of psychological disorders; an apparent 'cure' on the local level would only push them back into the sphere of the psyche.

Local treatment, however – relief of itching, inflammation, pain, etc. – is not neglected. By studying thoroughly the many medicinal plants growing in Tibet and its neighbouring countries, I found nearly two hundred plants to which the Asian has recourse for skin treatments. Hemp (*cannabis sativa*) seems to be the most frequently employed.

Central Asian healers obviously cannot deny the marvellous successes of modern dermatology but they claim that it commonly lacks wider perspectives.

The physician often manages to exert considerable influence on skin conditions by putting a check on *chu-ser* (lymph). His medical texts advise him to take care here 'to prevent the development of weak conditions'. A distinction must also be made between 'light' and 'dark' lymph. Whether this indicates substantial differences, or those only perceptible on the subtle level, is not mentioned in these texts, which in fact only very rarely make an explicit distinction between the two levels. Lymph is 'pale' when cold humours (i.e. air and/or phlegm) are in evidence, and 'dark' when hot bile or blood heated by bile are involved. Amongst the substances that restrict the production of pale lymph healers employ a Tibetan species of carrot, *piper longum*, a species of the pepper plant known as *Tsitraka* in Sanskrit, saffron and calamus. To diminish dark lymph, *asa foetida* and costus-root are used. The diet for excessive pale lymph includes *chang* (hot beer), veal, old butter (i.e. preserved for a long time), marmot-meat and horse-meat, whilst yoghurt and medicinal butter treated with sulphur are amongst the foods prescribed for dark lymph.

Yet another category of central Asian therapeutic methods involves the wearing of objects, to which certain curative effects are attributed by virtue of their emanations. Hence, in the case of goitre for example, apart from dispensing medicines and employing other methods, the healer quite commonly recommends wearing an otter skin around the neck. Healing properties are attributed to the emanations of precious and semi-precious stones: amber for eye complaints, turquoise (which is also often worn as jewellery) for liver complaints, coral for disorders of the blood vessels, and so on.

Whilst on the subject of Tibetan healing methods, I would like to point out that, as a general rule, it would not be advisable simply to pick 'goodies' out of the abundant wealth of Tibeto-Lamaist medical practice, with the intention of integrating them into one's own medical system. Many of these methods are only of relative value. Giving them due consideration and applying them appropriately requires a good knowledge of the entire Tibetan medical doctrine. This is a prerequisite for avoiding the dangers that could be provoked by exploiting isolated fragments out of context.

Such exploitations in essentially subtle domains appear to be especially dangerous. Long ago Edward Carpenter wrote: 'In all that science has ascertained, nothing seems more important to me than the fact that, if one shuts off thought and abides in that state, one eventually gains access to a sphere of consciousness which is situated beneath or behind thought and is utterly different from our normal level of consciousness'. But an Asian proverb says: 'The gods themselves cannot do anything to help a rogue'. When a patient is transported into these 'other levels of consciousness', that very material which has been suppressed and accumulated in the depths of his being, is uprooted and emerges on the surface from the 'primal depths within man'. One should bear in mind particularly that the transition to these 'other spheres' – whether undergone seriously or only nominally for therapeutic purposes – does not necessarily constitute a transition to true spirituality. René Guénon, amongst others, explained it like this: 'It is often only an inverted kind of spirituality; a path leading to the various retrogressive parodies of true spirituality. During the final period of an age undergoing a process of dissolution, most people have blocked the entrance to the higher spheres of spirituality. And having cut themselves off from them, the ultimate phase of their downfall ensues: the sluice-gates of pseudo-spirituality are opened from below and it is let loose upon mankind'.

At least for the central Asian, rooted as he is in a different conception of the world, it is on the whole perhaps less dangerous to come in contact with certain negative aspects of this 'world beyond', than it is for the modern Westerner. Many of the meditation states are more active for him than for other peoples of the world. But even for him it is not easy to contain the forces he uncovers in the sphere of the subconscious, to channel them constructively and integrate them into a truly spiritual framework. And the noblest and greatest people, of course, do not usually require any techniques in order to develop spiritually.

About Cancer

THE *gyu-shi*, a standard work of Tibetan medical literature, is considered a work with esoteric content – it is only
partly understood even by highly educated Tibetans. It
contains a long chapter dealing mainly with leprosy,
which is the key to several larger sections on mental illness. The secret correspondences characteristic of the diseases of 'destiny', which include both cancer and leprosy,
are considered to operate on an even more subtle level
than the equally elusive relationships between diseases of
widely differing organs. Examples of the latter include:
teeth and joints, the brain and certain functions of the
alimentary canal, the nasal cavity and mucous membranes
of the lower abdomen and so forth. Such relationships
have now occupied Western science for several decades,
but have always seemed self-evident to Tibetan doctors.

Cancer occurs far less frequently in central Asia than
in the West. This is probably due to the absence of a
whole series of precipitating factors in areas such as diet,
food preparation and processing, water supply, sex life,
mental and emotional states of tension which have been
aggravated by technological progress, and so on.

In the countries which border Tibet, the frequency of
cancer falls considerably below the world average. And in
Tibet itself it is almost certainly lower than that of a country like India.

Nevertheless, Tibetan texts have not neglected to examine this terrible affliction.

In the first chapter we mentioned the Tibetan division of disease into three areas of causation: the ordinary, the psychological and the fateful. Cancer belongs to the second and third types as far as the root causes are concerned. Environmental conditions, nutritional errors and so forth, only count as additional, precipitating factors.

An irritant, an 'extraordinarily pugnacious demonic poison', which is said to reside in the sick person's blood, is held responsible for the outbreak of cancer when conditions are ripe. Its 'astral colour'[1] is described as copper-red. It is stressed that the irritant is a remarkably 'subtle, minute agitator', far more difficult to perceive than others; this description is hardly ever applied to other illnesses in Tibetan medical works. One of its particularly nasty characteristics is the ability to disperse itself with lightning speed throughout the diseased person's blood, up to the head and into the legs. Parts of the body expressly stated in Tibetan medical works as possible targets for cancer tumours are: the head, the area of the throat, the stomach, the intestines, the skin, the joints, the musculature and the bones. I have not as yet found any information concerning lung cancer in Tibetan works, perhaps because it belongs to the forms of cancer hardly ever found in central Asia. It is well known that the sudden increase in lung cancer in the technologically advanced countries has led to campaigns against tobacco smoking. However, mice intensively exposed to tobacco smoke over long periods do not develop lung cancer, although they do develop skin cancer when smeared with carcinogenic substances. At first glance it also seems inexplicable, why, according to

[1] On the level of the second body, there is apparently a special colour spectrum which is to an extent similar to the physical one.

large-scale statistics, cigarette smokers are far more likely to develop lung cancer than pipe smokers. For researchers whose approach to the problem of cancer is similar to that of Tibetan men of learning, in that it takes account of psychological factors, the simple explanation is that the cigarette smoker is much more nervous than the pipe smoker and seems to be more subject to mental and emotional unrest. The conclusion of both Tibetan and psychosomatic medicine, is that states of stress and anxiety encourage and accelerate cancer.

According to Tibetan scholars, when the 'demonic poison' (virus) appears, the causes which precipitate the cancer produce a disturbance of those parts of the vitalizing second body which correspond to the parts of the body afflicted by the cancer. This disturbance also involves an interruption in the supply of the subtle counterpart of digested food. The overall disease of the blood, which manifests itself locally as a malignant tumour, is related to a break or short circuit in the 'vital current' caused by the cancerous cells. This is combined physically with an insufficient permeation of the organs by the 'breath'; and subtly, on the plane of the second body, with an inadequate circulation of *prana*, the Tibetan *srog-dzin*.

The more dense and physically coarse a human body is (a state which occurs especially when the afflicted person is motivated exclusively by material goals), the more difficult it is for the subtle essence of food to be propagated, as described earlier, throughout the second body. Tibetan scholars believe that the Western idea of the necessity for certain levels of calorie intake will be revised in the years or decades to come. It only enjoys such respect in the West because we are such a materially oriented civilization, the product of our technical development.

A general point that should be mentioned is the Tibetan view that when a tumour takes hold in the second body it does not necessarily mean that it is malignant, for non-malignant tumours also have their subtle equivalents.

What causes cancer? The Western specialist replies: cancer is an abnormal cellular growth which develops 'selfishly' regardless of the needs of the organism, and cancer cells can reach other parts of the body via the vascular system, and create additional cancer tissues. Whether the second part of this statement requires revision will be shown by the findings of cancer research over the next few years. Since operations on tumours which are performed too early sometimes appear to encourage the formation of metastases (cancerous tissues in other parts of the body), it is not impossible that in this respect another, as yet undiscovered, means of propagation is at work.

The central Asian healer views the aetiology of cancer in terms of a whole series of stratified causes, of which the final, direct precipitating factor is the 'poisonous demonic concentrate' (roughly: virus). Some Western cancer researchers are beginning to suspect that hitherto unknown viruses are the precipitating causes of cancer. The smallest known viruses today are so tiny that they can pass through porcelain and are only visible through an electron microscope. According to the Nobel prizewinner Professor W. M. Stanley, writing in 1956, the fact that we have not been able to detect viruses in cancer cells, does not by any means rule out the possibility of their existence. The extraordinarily tiny cancer precipitating virus described in Tibetan texts is possibly this very same long sought after carcinogen.

Various indications and symbolic representations concerning the onset of cancer suggest that a person tainted by his fate carries a cancerous disposition around in him for many years until one or more of the various cancer precipitating factors leads to the effective outbreak of the disease. This can take several decades depending on the circumstances. At the appearance of the final precipitating factor, a sort of 'vibratory infection' may even occur; this is the transference of a morbid vibration, due to 'decomposition' coming from the subtle level. This is possibly identical to the action described in Tibetan works, of the 'most potent, subtle, demonic poison'. As generally happens in the Lamaist healing art where subtle correspondences play a special role, the actual mechanics involved in the outbreak and cure of the disease are virtually impossible to define in habitual Western terms.

The psychological background to the origin and pathology of cancer is not particularly stressed in Lamaist medical works, probably because the connections are considered so obvious that to discuss them would be superfluous. This is the field to which quite a few renowned Western cancer researchers have begun to pay particular attention in recent years. A study was made of the mental characteristics of a large number of patients in the Veterans Administration Hospital in Long Beach, California. The personality structure of patients with carcinomas that had developed very quickly was compared with that of an equal number of patients whose tumours progressed extremely slowly. It was found in a large number of cases that, in the same environmental conditions and with the same methods of treatment, the more the mental disposition of the afflicted person was subject to psychological tension, the more malignant the cancer was.

Tibetan views concerning insufficient oxygen supply (in a sense, however, which extends beyond that which is purely measurable), coincide with the more recent results of Western research. Of interest also is the relationship between states of depression and tension and a marked reduction in the oxygen content of the blood, which has been confirmed by research in Canada according to information furnished by Professor T. G. Sleeswijk of Holland. All in all, the position of Tibetan medicine with regard to cancer – i.e. the relationship between cancer, oxygen deficiency and psychological factors – seems absolutely sound.

Diagnosis is of course easier in cases of skin cancer and surface tumours than in those of internal ones. This difficulty is obviously much more keenly felt by the average Tibetan healer than it is in the West, since he does not have access to our highly developed diagnostic aids. Some of the most skilled healers – roughly equivalent to the most distinguished category in the traditionally oriented Chinese medical profession – are said to be able to make a correct diagnosis 'on another level of consciousness', even where internal organs are concerned. The majority are exhorted to be on their guard, especially in regard to the distinction between malignant and non-malignant tumours. The *gyu-shi* stresses this point and states that it is especially difficult to grasp the nature of tumours when they are situated in fatty tissue.

Substances used in diagnostic tests appear to include even arsenic, which the doctor must use very skilfully of course, since the dose must be exactly suited to the purpose. (Just as with certain hormone preparations, arsenic also may stimulate or restrict the cancer according to the dosage.) Clinical collaboration between Asian healers and Western-style doctors could be useful in this field, especially if they were able to gain each other's confidence by virtue of their respective mental and human qualities.

Surgical interventions are not generally undertaken in the treatment of cancer in central Asia. Since the Tibetan physician regards cancer as the expression of a very grave malady which has secured a hold on the whole organism (including the second body), his attention is chiefly directed towards the treatment of the whole person. Where local surgical interventions are nevertheless advisable, cauterization is favoured. The areas of the body which can be treated in this way are of course much less numerous than those which can be dealt with by surgical operations. Where malignant tumours develop on the surface of the skin, a corresponding surface treatment is given – usually consisting of damp medicinal packs – during the general course of treatment.

The surface area of the part of the body under treatment in cancer must also be previously moistened when fumes of burning aromatic medicinal plants are applied. This, incidentally, is also virtually a universal rule for treating cancer in traditional Chinese medicine. Medicinal embrocations require likewise that the organs under treatment be moistened first.

As for medication, which is the subject of the following passage, it is frequently recommended that oral administration of medicines should be combined with the application of salves containing approximately the same medicaments. The salves used for this should, where possible, be heated before they are applied and then rubbed in.

On the subject of healing substances and diet requirements in cancer, an express warning is given against administering 'sweet' and 'white' medicines or 'sweet' and 'white' food or drink. The worst possible 'poison' in cancer is apparently refined white sugar.

Cancer patients are advised particularly to avoid sleeping during the day and excessive strain of any kind. In addition they should not 'ride on horseback', 'allow themselves to be carried away by any expression of anger', and on no account 'cross over running water'. Those afflicted by cancer are also counselled to 'drink pure water from mountain streams', in other words to avoid tap water.

I discussed the matter of the last mentioned rule with a Lamaist doctor some time ago. I was prompted to do so because of the ideas of a central European forestry official who had drawn wide support for his theories on hydraulics and water in general and had stressed the influence of 'healthy' and 'diseased' water in the West. In the view of authentic Tibetan physicians, 'bad' drinking water, even when it is well filtered and chemically purified, is undoubtedly a cancer precipitating factor. This obviously implies an effect at the level of the subtle body.

The Tibetan division of cancer into 'hot' and 'cold' types does not appear to me[2] clear enough for me to be able to enumerate here the medicaments recommended for these categories. I list only those which in all probability are indicated for virtually every type of cancer :

1. Musk. Apart from its other curative effects, it encourages nosebleeding (in the correct dosage, which can vary considerably from person to person). This is thought to be beneficial in cancerous conditions. However, I would advise Western cancer researchers to beware of imitations. Genuine musk was seldom found, even in Tibet where it originates.

2. Black sulphur. I have not as yet been able to identify this substance. It is either black mercuric sulphide, which

[2] Only the Tibetan linguist can guess the enormous difficulties involved here, especially in the symbolism of Tibetan medical works.

is mercury with sulphur rubbed into it – hence the black colour – or a black sulphur compound, possibly antimony sulphide.

3. Black incense. (A substance similar to olibanum, which has not yet been identified.)

The preceding remedies are mentioned in the *men-ngag-yon-ten-dyu-dyi-len-tab* and various standard medical works. Others also recommend aconite (to be administered with caution, naturally, because of its poisonous properties). Whether the latter can be used in all forms of cancer, is, as with many other recommended substances, not clearly ascertainable. According to a Protestant missionary, the Tibetans are said to prefer, for combating cancer, *aconitum ferrox* which comes mainly from Nepal. (*Aconitum* (*ferrox*) *Wall.* is one of the most poisonous types of aconite.) Tibetan and ancient Indian medicine also use it for leprosy. In Nepal, Sikkim, Assam and other areas near Tibet, no fewer than seventeen different types of aconite are to be found. These include *aconitum elwesie, aconitum chasmanthum, aconitum falconeri, aconitum heterophyllum, aconitum luridum, aconitum napellus, aconitum spicatum* and *aconitum palmatum*.

A species of juniper with thorns (possibly a variety of the Western juniper) is also sometimes recommended in the preparation of healing substances for treating cancer.

We have already mentioned that the psychiatric and non-psychiatric are very rarely completely separated in Lamaist medicine. The 'infinitesimal virus' mentioned at the beginning of this chapter, considered to be the direct precipitating element in cancer, is definitely linked with the influence of demons. Tibetan physiognomists also confirm this opinion.[3]

---

[3] The use of facial and ocular expression as a diagnostic aid is gener-

There is a strong indication that a close connection exists between the 'demonic poison' and the whole teaching of the fall of man and gradual corruption of the world, even though no specific reference is made to it in the Tibetan works mentioned in this book. The enlightened reader in the West is mistaken if he believes this to be merely an obscure sort of primitive superstition. What we find ourselves confronted with is an imposing cosmology containing a descriptive ontology right down to the finest detail. It incorporates mythology about the dissolution of a world paradise, which takes the form of a magnificent metaphysical drama, man being both actor and observer throughout. The Tibetan physician of high calibre, who has been instructed by a guru, possesses deep insights into this degeneration of the human race and into individual human destiny, in terms of a metaphysical field of force and the microcosm as a counterpart of the macrocosm.

A peculiarity of the Lamaist healing art is the way it combines curative procedures of a gross material nature with subtle factors that hardly seem connected to them. This also applies to the treatment of cancer in which the Tibetan healer employs particularly vigorous stomach massages, even when the cancer is located in a completely different part of the body. In this case he is acting on the 'submerged layers' of man which indirectly affect the organism as a whole. A Western equivalent of such practices, although much less effective, is the long-term administration recommended by some European healers, of coarse whole-meal bread to cancer patients.

---

ally regarded as a specialized science which is extremely difficult to learn. The specialists in question assert they can discern a 'demonic trait' in the eyes of most cancer cases, which is reminiscent of certain aspects of 'possession'.

The whole attitude of the Tibetan physician to the problem of cancer explains why our numerous experiments, especially with animals in which cancer is produced artificially, do not carry much weight with him. He is not to be dissuaded from the opinion that concern for the purely physical aspects of an evil rooted in deeper domains usually only leads to the creation of perpetually contradictory hypotheses. This holds true no matter how impressive the resources deployed or how monumental the intellectual effort.[4]

Nor has the central Asian healer failed to observe the relationship between cancer and the sexual function. He notes that failure of the sexual glands is nearly always combined with an increase in disposition towards swellings. He is probably also aware of the overproduction of hormones in the anterior lobe of the pituitary gland which occurs during the change of life of a woman. The attempts by various contemporary brain surgeons simply to remove a part of the pituitary gland in such cases, in order to curb the predisposition towards swellings, also belong, in his opinion, to the category of superficial techniques, which are a long way from tackling the malady at its roots.

The fact that cancer is rare amongst Tibetan monks who adhere to religious precepts, genuinely and not just for the sake of appearances, again demonstrates the con-

[4] Our Western cancer researchers are familiar with the maze of contradictions, completely unexpected results of experiments and inexplicable turns of events, which occur time after time in research work which is predominantly materially oriented. Hormones for instance – depending on the circumstances, the dose and whether they are male or female hormones – can either stimulate or combat cancer. Pioneers in medical science considered arsenic an invaluable aid in healing cancer centuries ago (providing it was used with extreme caution). On the other hand, it is thought to be the main cause of frequent cases of skin cancer in various parts of Argentina, where small quantities of it are present in the water supply (Dr. Tjebbo Franken, Holland).

nection between cancer and the sexual as well as the religious spheres. The sublimation of sexual energy – to use Western terminology – is regarded as an excellent preventive measure against cancer. On the other hand, sexual repression is said to be particularly conducive to it. A normal, healthy sex life is rated about halfway between the two. An important restraint, however, is that sexual intercourse with pregnant women, which is strongly felt to be against nature, is deemed to be a cancer producing factor which often only takes effect much later.

Certain yoga exercises also play a part in fighting and preventing cancer on 'subtler planes', because they reinforce the supply of *prana* which is the subtle counterpart of oxygen. The fight against cancer is thought to be enormously aided by the patient himself, principally by developing a vital attitude, and regarding the human organs, not as parts of a 'machine', but as 'animate entities'.

To conclude this chapter I would like to add that the most profound Lamaist scholars are of the opinion that even if Western research were able to find, as it did in the case of leprosy, really effective, practical and universally applicable healing methods for cancer, this would only be a momentary success – even though a very impressive one – since the root malaise would sooner or later become active elsewhere, possibly in the form of other, even more terrible diseases. For the Tibetan healer, the effective remedy for this 'original evil' lies within the sphere of religion. A description of the nature of this original evil which comes very close to the Tibetan view, was supplied by Thomas Carlyle when he pointed out that throughout the course of many centuries, the sum total of godlessness, lies and oppression of one man by his fellows, has ever increased. And each century has seen this undischarged debt of transgressions increase with renewed potency and passed on to those who followed.

But even in the light of this realisation, scholars and healers on a high level in Tibet, as elsewhere, are not diverted from the task of relieving the miseries of mankind whenever this can be done without running contrary to the aims of a higher order.

Mental Illness and Possession

THE SUCCESS rate of Tibetan methods in the treatment of mental illness is remarkable.

The highest ranking Tibetan physicians lead us to believe that the chief cause of severe mental derangement is to be found in the pursuit of a lifestyle which runs contrary to the inherent disposition of the afflicted person and his spiritual destiny. In serious cases there remains, for the highest spiritual aspects of the patient, no alternative but detach themselves from him, leaving the remaining layers of his personality to their fate. This process is, in a sense, comparable to death – a living death.

As readers who know something about Indian and Tibetan cosmology are probably aware, man is considered to be an aggregate of 'vehicles' (*skandha* in ancient Indian philosophy and *pung-po* in the Tibetan). In traditional Chinese cosmology too we find similar concepts, the difference being that the proposed number of 'component parts' is larger in most schools. After death, these vehicles or component parts of man are dismantled by varying degrees according to set laws.

The highest spiritual principle (i.e. very roughly what the Christian regards as the soul) is not counted as a component part of this vehicle aggregate. Most Buddhists – there are no less than eighteen different principal sects in

Tibet alone – avoid precise definitions of this highest spiritual principle, whereas they devote detailed description and speculation to the various vehicles of the aggregate.

To prevent misunderstandings, I would emphasize here that this withdrawal of the soul which features in Tibetan psychiatry, is somewhat different from so-called 'spiritual death'. The latter is the definitive, negative separation of the highest spiritual principle from the lower levels of man, which Tibetan and classical Indian philosophy describe as an irrevocable descent to the 'depths of hell', from which it is impossible to rise again. Spiritual death is considered extremely rare; it is the final stage of a fully conscious and persistent pursuit of evil, to which 'Forgive them Lord, for they know not what they do!' no longer applies. The details of this awesome spiritual catastrophe are treated as top-secret teachings.

There is a second category of mental illness, which applies to an incomparably greater number of cases. According to Tibetan thought – expressed in Western concepts – it originates in a discordant interaction of vehicles in the vehicle aggregate of man. As a rule, this is associated with a displacement of the layers of personality of which the integrated self is normally composed. This interference is either permanent or confined to longer or shorter periods of time. Depending on the presence or temporary retreat of interfering vehicles, the afflicted person experiences changes in consciousness. When this is accompanied by confusion in the patient's vehicle aggregate, the result is the kind of split in consciousness which the Western psychiatrist encounters in schizophrenia. In less serious cases interference can sometimes be eliminated by shock therapy, which arouses the displaced vehicle as it were and calls it back to its natural place. As long as no definitive and irrevocable separation has occurred, a displaced vehicle remains attached to the afflicted person by means of a 'cord' composed of the subtle matter of the second body.

The methods of shock therapy, adopted from traditional Indian ones, do not of course include ECT (electro-convulsive therapy). However, there are certainly equivalents, such as bringing the patient news (untrue) of his mother's sudden death, or unexpectedly pouring painfully hot water over him.

A 'displacement of vehicles' is thought to be caused by the disintegration of the vehicle aggregate, which is conducive to the occupation of component parts of the personality by vehicles from outside. A factor which apparently encourages this process, is the practice of hypnosis or offering oneself for hypnosis experiments. When disintegration is caused in this way, the result is not necessarily experienced during the same lifetime. Hence, a predisposition towards schizophrenia can often be traced back to 'inherited' tendencies – though not in the usual sense. Various states of intoxication, including alcoholic inebriation and those induced by narcotics, are also conducive to a disintegration of the vehicle aggregate.

The successful cures which some psychiatrists claim to have attained by using hypnotic techniques are regarded as transient successes by central Asian healing practitioners who are well versed in the subject. Not only in the psychiatric field, but also in a very general sense, they tend to believe that, in the sphere of healing, the very cures which appear so strikingly prompt are those which have to be paid for by damage which often only sets in years later or in a subsequent incarnation.

The vehicles which take possession of a part of the

human personality from without are called 'spectres' or 'demons' by the ordinary Tibetan.[1] The scholar, however, regards them as mental entities or projections (mostly of a lower order), or as psychic fields of force, either natural or contrived. The way they are classified in Tibetan psychiatry is not unlike Paracelsus' scheme. Hence there are vehicles from various mental-spiritual levels – those which stem from the decaying vehicle aggregate of dead people and those 'contrived' ones which owe their origin either to an act of will exercised by a malicious person, or to consciously or unconsciously transmitted thought forms and mass psychoses on the human level.

In the West too there are manifestations which the Tibetan would unhesitatingly put under the heading of possession. Crimes, for instance, for which the perpetrator often cannot supply any motive at all. The Tibetan scholar would even include here such mild forms as the case reported recently in the West of five youths, the youngest of whom was fifteen years old, who stole half a dozen cars one after the other and abandoned them when the petrol had run out. By their chaotic driving, they caused a long succession of serious accidents. When questioned after their arrest about the reason for this behav-

---

[1] Tibetan demonology divides the vehicles related to states of possession into several hundred main categories, with numerous subdivisions.

According to Tibetan translations of ancient Indian texts, there are particular vehicles (demons) which 'take someone over' especially if he violates religious laws, lives alone in an otherwise unoccupied house, and so on.

On my travels, I found that similar notions also exist in remote parts of Iceland, amongst other places.

In cases of schizophrenia, the Tibetan healer, like the ancient Indian physician, must first ascertain by studying the symptoms just what type of demons have seized upon the sick person. The specialist can then often discover the rhythm in which the energy of the invading vehicle rises and falls, and choose the time for action accordingly.

iour, they declared that whilst committing the offence they had been 'under the influence of speed intoxication'!

Like the Tibetan's, other cosmologies which are non-material oriented also expound many states of possession. They hold that especially people with a disposition towards mediumship – because their astral bodies are more susceptible to outside influences – easily become dominated by foreign 'entities'. The latter infiltrate their astral bodies and either partially or completely displace and inhibit the rightful 'inhabitant'. Just as in Tibetan cosmology, they also include a great variety of entities in this category: 'elements' of the dead which await their opportunity to become manifest, certain 'vibrations' from living people and various other higher and lower invisible entities.

Tibetan views on this subject correspond in many respects to ancient Indian concepts. They distinguish approximately twenty different influences, even amongst the simplest types of demonic possession. These range from entities which occupy higher psychical spheres to spectres of a lower order.

The behaviour of the entity involved is reflected in the whole conduct of the possessed person. Its most salient characteristics should be familiar to the demonologist. One type can be recognised by the fact that the person it possesses becomes irascible, proud, malicious and pompous, and suddenly develops an extraordinarily intense craving for meat and strong alcohol. Another category engenders a crooked, swaying walk, a staring look, very red eyes and also a sudden, unusually strong craving for honey, sweetmeats and milk.

When treating splits in consciousness, the Tibetan healer not only attaches importance to removing the influences which have penetrated the patient, he also stresses the general strengthening of his powers of resistance. This involves the selection of a suitable diet and the administration of medicines.

Because they break down into such numerous major and minor categories, the study of these influences is a very extensive branch of Tibetan psychiatry. In the first of five groups of mental illness involving possession – which are mentioned later – there are no less than eighteen different main categories of such influences! The magical cosmology of the Tibetan gives him recourse to interventions which amount to either chasing out or pacifying demonic influences. The more practice healers of distinction have in this field, the more they seem to reach the conclusion that it is much more difficult to tackle an evil at its roots than to remove symptoms and momentarily expel demons, which amounts to a sort of Tibetan equivalent of the Western 'instantaneous success'.

In strengthening the patient's general power of resistance, especially that of the mentally sick, a good, conscientious Tibetan doctor regards the prescription of an invigorating diet and tonics simply as a transitional stage. During this period he tries to influence the psychological level of the patient suffering from splits in consciousness at the earliest opportunity, by taking advantage of his lucid moments.

Instances of preventive 'expulsion of spectres' also occur where a person's whole environment is allegedly conducive to mental illness and 'poisoning' and therefore renders him vulnerable to demonic influences – or more correctly, to dangerous psychic fields of force. This also plays a role in child psychiatry. A strongly recommended prophylactic for demonic child illnesses is to avoid startling or frightening children. The latter is considered quite criminal since it renders them far more easily accessible to demonic influences, 'in proportion to the consequences of the burden of sin accumulated in previous lives'.

Apart from the two important categories of mental diseases mentioned above, there are also those which have specific causes such as injuries, infections and so forth.

Since the Tibetan art of healing – and Tibetan science as a whole – emphasizes taking account of and understanding a wider context and its all-inclusive correlations, it avoids specific compartmentalising. The scientist, for instance, who at a congress or seminar demands that an Asian scholar should 'speak more to the point', brands himself as very close to a barbarian in the eyes of the latter, and proves that he has not the faintest idea about the attitude of Asian scholars towards scientific matters. And this applies even more in Tibetan psychiatry, since it is intimately interwoven with nearly every other sphere of Lamaist medicine. This interrelationship goes so far that there are hardly any psychiatrists as such in the 'Forbidden Land'. It is expected that virtually every Lamaist doctor should have a thorough knowledge of psychiatry.

This is clearly reflected throughout their medical literature. It is, moreover, even more difficult than in other areas of Tibetan medicine to demarcate what is specifically psychiatric from what is not. References to psychiatric matters are found in chapters where least expected, whilst chapters exclusively or principally allocated to psychiatry are very few. The third part of the *gyu-shi*, for instance, which is divided into more than ninety chapters, contains only five consecutive chapters designated as primarily psychiatric in content. And the fifth and last of these goes into seemly non-psychiatric domains to such a degree, that even a Westerner well acquainted with the Tibetan language would at first regard it as non-psychiatric. In a completely different part of the *gyu-shi* again, there is another chapter like this, not easy to find, the content of which is predominantly psychiatric. References to mental disturbances of various kinds are also to be found scattered throughout other chapters.

In explicitly psychiatric texts, not only in the *gyu-shi*, a striking division occurs – child psychiatry is dealt with separately.

Whereas disturbances caused by the penetration of alien vehicles into the patient constitute by far the majority of adult mental illnesses, its incidence is so great amongst children that Tibetan child psychiatry virtually only encompasses the treatment of such disturbances. Indeed, central Asians take the view that children are particularly vulnerable to the dangers of demonic influences. It is possible, however, for the mother to contribute significantly during pregnancy to warding off these evil influences, by taking special care to have only 'good and pure thoughts', which of course contributes much more to routing out demons than any kind of external practice. At the time immediately following birth, the child's 'burden of sin' carried over from earlier lives again plays a definite role. This burden of sin determines, in proportion to the child's slowly emerging mental-spiritual mould and the positive or negative aspects of his so-called vibrations, whether he will repel or, as is far more often the case, attract demons.

For the Tibetan scientist of a particularly scholarly turn of mind, the Tibetan translation of the ancient Indian *Kumara-Tantra* presents a very good though somewhat primitive description of child psychiatry. On studying its contents, one is struck especially by the idea that the odour of mentally disturbed children, regarded as a symptom, is purported to provide essential keys as to the nature of the disturbance.

Generally speaking – not only in relation to the psychiatric treatment of children – the burning of incense and exorcism play an important role in overcoming mental illnesses caused by invading vehicles (i.e. 'possession' or 'demonic' influences'). In addition, they administer medications, including a large variety of substances harmless in themselves which to my knowledge have not yet been employed, even experimentally, in any Western clinics. It should however be possible for the Western psychiatrist, who not only has command of specialist knowledge but is also in a position to win the confidence of traditional Asian healers on the intellectual-spiritual level, to add a considerable number of valuable new healing substances to the extant pharmacopoeia of Western psychiatry as a result of such contact. This has indeed already been achieved in at least one instance with the introduction of the so-called 'lunatic weed' or serpent wood, *rauwolfia*.

The formulae and incantations employed in exorcism are based on precepts and experience which go back hundreds of years – and even thousands in the case of those adopted from the ancient indigenous *Bon* cult. Nevertheless, I believe that if we were to take up similar practices in the West, certain incantations such as those which for instance the time-honoured ritual of the Roman Catholic Church is in a position to offer, might prove to be better suited to the character and needs of Western man than Lamaist ones. When it comes to incorporating the religious sphere, the Westerner does not, of course, require specifically Tibetan impulses.

The incantations used in Tibetan psychiatry consist mostly of series of syllables which have been taken straight from ancient Indian Sanskrit texts. According to information passed to me orally by Tibetan healers, the recitation of these incantations depends primarily on what mental images the healer combines with them as they are uttered. Intonation also plays an important role which may not, on principle, be rigidly documented, but must be personally taught to select pupils by a teacher who is called to the task (to be handed on later to others of the same calling). In the hands of a scholar who does not have the benefit of such 'living instruction', even the cream of Sanskrit incantation formulae are held to be completely worthless.

It is rather extraordinary that the Tibetans, who possess a language which is noted in many parts of Asia for its magical properties, seldom recite incantation texts in Tibetan. In its pronunciation, for example, the Tibetan language distinguishes three different tones, each of which is said to deploy its own particular influence on the subtle level. Some sounds are pronounced with the tongue between the teeth. They are produced almost exclusively by the lips and the oral cavity. These sounds correspond to the air humour. Then there are strongly aspirated sounds, the formation of which requires the participation of a larger area of the organism. They correspond to bile, or the energetic principle. A third category is an undulating sound and it seems to come from the innermost depths of the body. The organs used to produce them extend right into the abdomen. These sounds correspond to phlegm or the material principle. The fact that the main seat of phlegm is not located in the lower part of the body, is, to the Tibetan way of thinking, not contradictory. The relatively rare incantation formulae recited in the Tibetan language are usually intoned at a particularly low pitch.

According to the ideas expressed in the most important psychiatric traditions in Tibeto-Lamaist medicine, as laid down in the *tso-we-tse-yi-pag-sam-jon*, the book designated 'king of medical works', the majority of vehicles under the heading of demonic influences can be divided into the following five categories:

1. The *jung-po* class (roughly: psychic fields of force interwoven with the effects of the four elements – water, fire, earth and air).

2. *Nyo* producing. By *nyo* the Tibetan understands a sort of goading or stimulation of the senses, which gives rise to disturbances of consciousness. The states of inebriation caused by alcohol consumption or unbridled sexual passion also belong to this category.

3. Vehicles which drain a person of his ability to concentrate and in the worst cases completely rob him of his memory.

4. Vehicles connected with planetary influences. These are regarded as the direct cause of epilepsy.

5. The influence of entities which Tibetan science designates as *lu* and the ancient Indian as *naga*. They are the origin of the most serious mental diseases, and also of leprosy, and not only the type which attacks the nervous system. Generally speaking, a relatively close connection is said to exist between psychological phenomena and pathological skin conditions.

From the above mentioned categories, let us now take the example of possession caused by *nyo* producing demons. Infiltration by the latter into a person's vehicle aggregate is encouraged by excessive grief and anguish, which are considered the direct causes. This is sometimes bound up with factors which stem from specific character traits, nutritional errors and so on. The disease is divided into seven different types according to which factors directly precipitate it: (1) overall prevalence of air, (2) of bile, (3) of phlegm, (4) excess of all three humours, (5) mental states of worry and depression, (6) 'poisons', (7) causes which are connected with the patient's individual disposition. In each one of these seven subdivisions the most important symptoms are recounted. In the sixth category, poisons, for instance, these consist of a marked diminution of the radiance emanating from the face and eyes, and a general lowering of energy, and confusion in the patient's mental and emotional worlds. In each category, the most important methods of treatment and medications recommended for administration are also mentioned. An example: in the second category, prevalence of bile, the patient first undergoes cleansing cures using five different medicines; then follows the administration of a mixture of seven medicaments in powder form; bloodletting in the region of the heart; administration of, and simultaneous lubrication of the skin with, medicinal butter treated with gentian; plus a prescribed diet which includes veal and other varieties of fresh meat. Treatment of the fifth category emphasizes the influence on the psychological factors. The most essential part is played here by particularly 'affectionate treatment' and very personal, individual care of the patient. In other words, precisely that which, with the best will in the world, the well organised 'machinery' of modern Western medical establishments is hardly in a position to offer.

As already mentioned, the Tibetan healer includes epilepsy in that category of diseases involving intruding vehicles associated with planetary influences. These vehicles temporarily, and in a violent manner, overpower a portion of the vehicle aggregate of people whose disposition provokes such invasions. According to various medical works, epileptic fits usually occur on eight precisely specified days of the thirty day Tibetan month : the fourth, eighth, eleventh, fifteenth, eighteenth, twenty-second, twenty-fifth and twenty-ninth. It would be interesting to discover whether Western specialists have also established a similar rhythmical frequency of epileptic fits on particular days.

As in the ancient Indian works from which this knowledge derives, cases of epilepsy where the sick person becomes very thin, arches his eyebrows, rolls his eyes and is subject to especially violent convulsions, are considered extraordinarily difficult, if not impossible, to cure.

Strangely enough, I was unable to find any description of multiple sclerosis in Tibetan psychiatric texts. In the West this disease is rather widespread.[2] Since it is estimated that sixty per cent of all cases of multiple sclerosis throughout the world are under treatment in two countries, the USA and Germany, whilst the population of the two only comprises roughly ten per cent of the earth's population, it could be that it is a disease of civilisation which has not yet afflicted the Tibetans.

The extraordinarily long chapter which concludes the predominantly psychiatric passages in the *gyu-shi*, is a so-called esoteric chapter and is among the most difficult to understand in Tibetan literature. Its style is so symbolic in places that only those with the most expert knowledge of the language and spiritual life of central Asia can glimpse the import of its contents. And even they, for want of equivalents in Western terminology and thought processes, can only proffer an approximation. Those who can only grasp the apparent meaning will perhaps con-

[2] The 1971 figure for England and Wales is 6,356. (Tr.)

sider this chapter totally non-psychiatric, even though it is referred to as explicitly psychiatric in a synopsis provided in the same book.

Derived from the concept of a progressive degeneration of humanity which is taken for granted by Tibetan science, it begins with a description of a state of depravity set in remotest antiquity. By dint of the folly, greed and 'horrifying thoughts' of most people – who were, moreover, not open to teaching – the 'substance' of this patient earth was increasingly impaired. The perpetually increasing burden of sin, together with its related consequences, is said to have increased beyond measure the number of vehicles which threatened men with possession. In conjunction with erroneous lifestyle and eating habits, it apparently also led to a general state of disharmony of the humours. This is said to have manifested in the appearance of the 'unbearable' and awesome disease of leprosy, amongst other things. With regard to diagnosis in this context, a threefold division into 'ordinary', 'inner' and 'occult' diagnosis occurs, which is at variance with the diagnostic methods for individual diseases put forward in most other chapters. What is remarkable is that diagnosis based on the patient's reaction to certain key medications in fact belongs to the sphere of occult diagnosis and not to the ordinary type, as might be expected. This concerns a 'reversal of correspondences', which should at least make sense to someone familiar with the main principles of medieval alchemy.

In the following passages too, the Tibetan author's trains of thought lead repeatedly into esoteric domains. This can be seen in the passage which stresses that not only in certain cases of leprosy but also in serious mental disorders considered as diseases of destiny, even the most useful and far-reaching procedures can only succeed if the patient's individual destiny, which is subject to a higher order of justice, favours it.

Strange though it may seem to the Western scientist, the Tibetans believe that there is an intimate connection between serious mental illness on the one hand, and formidable infirmities like leprosy on the other. In ancient Chinese text books the appellation *feng* is used for paralysis, leprosy and mental illness alike! 'Forceful cures' are viewed from this standpoint as effecting but a displacement of the evil which lies dormant in the depths of the person's being, either in the same or in an ensuing incarnation.

The continuing increase of nervous and mental disorders in the West prompted me recently to compare notes on this important question with central Asian scientists. Contrary to expectation, they are not of the opinion that this marked increase is attributable to excessive demands on nervous resources and other consequences of the capricious blessings of progress. This may seem odd at first glance, but they believe that by 'fighting diseases on the surface level' – diseases, that is, which people have brought upon themselves by misdeeds committed in this and in previous lives – a transference of the 'basic evil' to other areas can occur. One of the men with whom I corresponded writes: 'You have eradicated nearly all infectious diseases and achieved the fantastic in the field of surgical technology. The "root evil", which lies beyond the material sphere, is not, however, eliminated by such means and in time surfaces elsewhere like a water course issuing forth from a hillside when other exits have been blocked. So the increase in nervous and mental illnesses and the incidence of cancer should not come as a surprise to you'. Such observations are not the products of eccentrics but of men regarded as learned and wise who have achieved notable success in many fields, including psychiatry.

It is clear that in the most crucial areas the central Asian scholar is continually aware of the connection with the religious sphere. This was indeed once the general case in the Christian West too, in a form which corresponded to Western cosmology. In the course of time, 'self-adulation', encouraged by technological progress, has wrenched us further and further away from these spiritual domains. Hence, to Tibetan sages firmly anchored in religion, we in the West are fundamentally tending to take into account only 'instantaneous successes'.

To return again to unusual aspects of Tibetan psychiatry, I would like to include here the fact that even in serious forms of mental disturbance, the medicines dispensed are often very simple and in many cases not specifically Tibetan. I know from experience and experiment, hitherto on a very small scale to be sure, that the Tibetan healer, by skilfully and carefully compounding simple and, in themselves, completely harmless substances – the procedure for which is nevertheless based on extensive experience – can cause beneficial 'agitation' in the patient's consciousness of an intensity hardly conceivable in other parts of the world.

Turning now to the nursing and care of mental patients, they are not usually treated in special medical institutions, and this puts a heavy burden on their family and environment. It is believed that the vibrations which emanate from people suffering from mental disturbances would very soon 'contaminate' a psychiatric clinic. Doctors treating them must therefore also learn, first and foremost, how to shield themselves and their assistants from these radiations. This is not achieved – as some Westerners seem to believe – by doing yoga exercises 'like a steam engine'! Certain substances, such as precious stones, are amongst the influences purported to act as 'disinfectants' in such circumstances. At all events, it is interesting to note that various Western psychiatrists also attest that they have noticed the influence of environmental factors of this nature. I recall at least one case of a psychiatrist stating that under some pretext he sometimes advised patients who seemed to be threatened by emanations to change their surroundings. Just imagine how far Hahnemann, for instance, might have come if he had not had the courage to stand by his medicines publicly, but had dispensed them instead 'under some pretext' as 'distilled water'!

In many respects the central Asian healer has a much easier job than his Western colleague when treating mental diseases; especially when they are related to the sexual sphere. For various reasons, such cases are less abundant than in the West, but not too rare nonetheless. The Tibetan doctor is in a much more favourable situation because the patient (in his 'lucid' moments), and the people around him, quite bluntly tell the doctor the whole truth. This they do without the conscious – or, what is often even more difficult, unconscious – inhibitions which, by giving a distorted picture of the true state of affairs, would impede the doctor's treatment and the healing process. Cases interwoven with the sexual sphere are considered particularly difficult when the disturbance in psychological balance originates in the patient attempting to penetrate spiritual spheres, whilst continuing to surrender to his sensual instincts, or forcibly suppressing them, instead of – to put it in Western terms – sublimating them from within. Tibetan medicine believes that in cases like this, it is often only the minister who can now be of any assistance and, as frequently happens in Tibet, this implies the minister within the doctor! Many Tibetan scholars seem to be of the opinion, incidentally, that even performing simple yoga exercises, whether for curative or other purposes, necessitates total sexual abstinence.[3]

In concluding this chapter, I would like to make the additional point that when considering possible collaboration between Western psychiatrists and Tibetan healers with a great deal of experience in the psychiatric field, it will be important to be clear as to what is to be designated 'normal' and 'abnormal'. It is well known that central Asian and Western assessments are worlds apart in this respect. A man who consistently overworks himself simply to raise his standard of living, and then collapses in the prime of life from overwork, is regarded as completely normal by us — amongst learned Tibetans, however, as abnormal. By contrast, many Tibetans consider it absolutely normal for someone to devote himself to particularly arduous practices for ten years, merely so that he at last reaches the stage where he can sit naked in the depths of winter throughout an entire night and keep from freezing to death by means of certain imaginary pictures. Most Westerners, on the other hand, would not only think him abnormal but definitely certifiable! One will therefore first have to establish norms in this and similar respects, in

---

[3] Since my prime concern in this book is to introduce what is unfamiliar to the West, I only touch on what is already familiar insofar as seems necessary for an understanding of the whole picture. I have therefore refrained from giving an outline of the various yoga exercises, which are well known anyway, thanks to a large number of books and so forth on the subject. Tibetan healing methods include yoga exercises. They are not, however, concerned with the level of being closest to the divine, but with that which verges directly upon it.

order to be able at least to converse together. This will require considerable tolerance on both sides, since in setting up standards to define 'normal' and 'abnormal', a certain amount of arrogance – and occasionally even opportunism – usually develops. And even within a single culture, widely differing norms often co-exist. What is considered good and completely normal in one century can later be regarded as bad and sometimes even as criminal!

The 'complexes' of the Tibetan, moreover, also take on a different dimension from ours. It is clear therefore, that collaboration with learned central Asians, particularly in the psychiatric field, requires not only specialized knowledge and personal qualities commensurate with the level of culture from which they stem, but also exceptionally wide and generous intellectual horizons.

Co-operation between Western and Tibetan Doctors

THE BRILLIANT results of modern medicine should not blind us to the gloomy side of the picture. The struggle with many diseases is still in vain or else shows very modest positive results. Millions suffer from malignant forms of virtually incurable diseases of the joints. Countless numbers in those very countries which are most technologically advanced suffer from severe neuroses and, in spite of the tremendous resources allocated to the fight against cancer, it is still spreading. Today[1] in England and Wales, for example, every fifth death is caused by cancer.

Since medicine has increasingly acknowledged psychosomatic interaction in health and disease, the impetus towards a new medical orientation has grown appreciably. It is now certain that the psyche influences the pathogenesis of stomach and intestinal ulcers, just as acute kidney infections and high blood pressure can be influenced by bringing about a mental change in the patient. As a result, more attention is being directed towards hitherto little known healing arts which have a reputation for success, such as the Tibetan and the traditional Chinese.

Until recently, work with Tibetan healing practitioners was accompanied by inordinate difficulties, due to the

[1] 1971. (Tr.)

country's great geographical isolation.[2] In China on the other hand, Western doctors and traditional Chinese healers frequently came into close contact decades ago. This occurred because rich Chinamen, following the motto that 'two heads are better than one', sometimes underwent treatment at the hands of a Western doctor and a Chinese healer simultaneously. When this happened, however, it was often a case of competition rather than genuine co-operation. If, for instance, on the basis of the complex pulse diagnosis alone – discussed elsewhere in this book – the Chinese healer claimed that the patient was suffering from a disease of a vital organ, indicated by irregularities in the respective pulse zones, then it was always possible for the rich Chinese patient to have this diagnosis verified immediately by his Western-style doctor using the newest diagnostic aids of Western medical science.

In spite of the growth of technology and the gradual elimination of hindrances to travel in the 'Forbidden Land' it was exceedingly difficult to make contact with authentic Asian healers in Tibet itself, even before it was occupied by the Chinese.[3] It can be seen from occasional allusions to the treatment of disease in the travel reports of many foreign authors and of experts of long-standing that they did not once have the opportunity of meeting a single genuine healer. Even in the case of genuinely cultured Westerners who possess the necessary tact and sensitivity to associate with an Asian élite, the 'real' Asian healer somehow senses their inner scepticism and withdraws himself. And even when, as an exception, a Westerner has gained their confidence, he sooner or later runs the risk of

---

[2] Since the Chinese occupation it is, of course, even more difficult to enter Tibet. (Tr.)

[3] In the early 1950's. (Tr.)

putting his relationship with Tibetan scholars to the test, by dint of his great curiosity – which would be completely justified to the Western way of thinking – concerning so-called esoteric spheres in Lamaist medicine. All this is, of course, based on the prerequisite that he has a good command of the Tibetan language.

The possibilities today of making contact with Tibetan physicians have multiplied.[4] Theoretically it should even be possible to bring one or more Lamaist doctors to the West.[5] An important prerequisite for co-operation would be our ability to convince the eminent Tibetan healer that collaboration with him is justified – even necessary – in view of higher spiritual considerations. Material attractions have no power over people who practise their profession in a genuinely dedicated fashion.

We Westerners have for years been more clearly observed by central Asians than most Europeans and Americans would deem possible. All our activities and goings-on, the 'demon' technology, the constantly increasing current of 'evil' thoughts[6] and much more of a similar nature, do not escape their attention. This does not require a telepathic means of communication, as many would believe, because for years it has been possible, even in Tibet, to procure news through ordinary channels. In the years following the Second World War, the modern Tibetan press (various newspapers and a monthly journal distributed in

[4] This statement was made before the advent of the Chinese. Contact with such Tibetan healers is to some extent still possible, for instance in Nepal and India. (Tr.)

[5] I heard recently that a Tibetan Lama, resident in London, is planning to do just this. (Tr.)

[6] I once read a letter written to a minister-physician describing the terrible damage which had occurred in a European town as a result of the war, to which he replied, "It is simply the materialisation of human thoughts!"

the border areas) had soon invented an extensive and appropriate specialized vocabulary to describe the most varied aspects of our Western civilisation.

These people are even aware of our greatest tragedy – that an inexorable fate has put a tremendous source of power, which demands a very high degree of maturity if it is not to be turned against humanity, into the hands of people, who as a species are extremely immature. And whilst our technical science creates ever increasing riches and more and more stupendous educational possibilities, it cannot prevent the fact that this abundance of economic and intellectual wealth exists alongside widespread moral impoverishment, indeed, depravity. Central Asian sages, and amongst them healers of the highest calibre, regard our nuclear fission particularly as an 'interference with the workings of a higher order' – and not only nuclear fission for war purposes! Not only hydrogen bomb explosions, about which such a storm of protest has been raised, but also peacetime atomic piles, produce increasing radiation fallout. This forms deposits in the bones which last for decades. Are they justified, these exceptional people ask themselves, in publicly proclaiming the whole of their knowledge in order to put God's creatures back on their feet – creatures moreover who continually and increasingly defy a 'higher justice' to their own detriment? And if an 'atomic death' of unimaginable proportions should set in as a reprisal for such behaviour, might not their secrets offer perhaps the last remaining possibility for producing a means of defence? They could not put such knowledge at the disposal of the West unless the survival of a portion of a humanity so set in its self adulation were really desired by this 'higher order'.

The more the genuine sage believes he has access to so-called inner spaces, the more he experiences the burden of an awesome responsibility – a responsibility not restricted to the human sphere only.

As soon as authentic healers are moved to co-operate, efforts to respond could be furthered in the following way. Westerners who feel they have a vocation for the task could devote themselves to the study of modern Western medicine and the Tibetan language, and go to Tibet[7] to carry out the undertaking. There they would endeavour to gain the confidence of eminent healers by virtue of their spiritual and intellectual standing. It is important that they should not lose touch with modern Western medicine or the intellectual and religious foundations of the West during their stay in central Asia, since only he who can remain grounded in his own philosophy is equal to the immense task of bridging the gulf between two cultures! Attempts to bait the Tibetans by becoming converted to Lamaism or the like would simply be considered laughable amongst the central Asian élite.

In order to explore the possibilities of effective co-operation with Lamaist physicians, a seminar, which was on principle open to both members and non-members of the medical profession, was held in a central European town in 1955. It was clear from the outset that any attempt to bring together two such widely differing medical philosophies faced enormous difficulties, since they are based on totally divergent intellectual-spiritual assumptions. So much so that even the Lamaist doctor's sensory perceptions, which play such a critical part in diagnosis, do not always correspond precisely with those of the Western doctor. In addition, a rapprochement of the two sys-

[7] Now no longer possible. They could, however, go to India or Nepal. (Tr.)

tems is fraught with almost overwhelming linguistic and practical problems.

In the course of the seminar it unfortunately became clear that older doctors, including a European psychiatrist who was interested in exploiting central Asian medicine, took the standpoint that those well acquainted with traditional Asian healing arts should themselves first become Western-style doctors before being allowed to discuss medicine with Western doctors! This none too generous approach understandably reaped its just rewards. It is known that the Tibetan doctor must study for up to twenty years before he is even considered of any use as a doctor by Tibeto-Lamaist standards. Neither would any serious-minded person well acquainted with the Tibetan healing art lower himself to dance attendance upon any Western system.

A few months later, the news came from China that the Chinese medical council[8] had decided to give equal recognition to serious traditional healing practitioners and to doctors with diplomas from Western universities – or universities equipped according to modern Western principles. It was also decided to incorporate them as fully qualified members of the Chinese medical profession.

When China could no longer stave off Western knowledge and modern industrialisation, there was a tendency at first to take the accepted Asian traditions, together with the knowledge which Asian scholars and sages had acquired over thousands of years, and throw it all overboard. Whereas in present-day India,[9] for example, many scientists still take this attitude, it appears that in China ever widening circles are coming to the conclusion that though

---

[8] Or the Chinese equivalent of the General Medical Council. (Tr.)
[9] 1957.

a scientist must initially be equipped with a sceptical attitude, this scepticism becomes exaggerated and destructive if it disregards the undeniable facts. Ancient Chinese knowledge has been increasingly drawn upon for some time now, especially in cases where it is believed that modern Western medicine is not in a position to do very much. But it is obvious that the Chinese are astute enough to derive benefit from the many advantages which our modern Western medicine has to offer.

During the years between the two World Wars, it was at times declared illegal in China to practise medicine based on traditional Chinese principles – legislation which, by the way, caused spasmodic, stormy public protests. Now, on the other hand, a National Academy for Research into Ancient Chinese Medicine has been set up, as well as large clinics for trying it out. The study of traditional Chinese medicine was incorporated into the syllabus of numerous medical faculties as early as 1957, and there are reports that since 1956, many thousands of Chinese doctors have enthusiastically been studying the contents of ancient Chinese medical books.

It should now, therefore, be clear to many leading Chinese, that collaboration between Western-style Chinese doctors and Lamaist healers could in many cases also lead to results as effective as those achieved by co-operation with tradition-oriented Chinese healers. The awareness, however, that Lamaist medicine is much more difficult than the ancient Chinese to separate from religious factors, acts as a drawback. In spite of this, given the uncanny talent of the Chinese – metaphorically speaking – to 'mix fire with water', it is still possible that such collaboration will sooner or later be instigated from the Chinese side. At all events, the prospect is far too tempting for the Chinese, who are no doubt clever enough not to go on shelving the idea indefinitely because of certain doctrinal attitudes. Besides, a rapprochement of the Lamaist medical profession and other healing systems[10] is possible on more than one level.

During the completion of the second half of this book, incidentally, I had unexpected opportunity to reflect upon one aspect of such co-operation in a very personal way. Just after finishing the section on Tibetan demonology, by a strange 'accident' I broke my foot. The mishap occurred as the result of a singular chain of events during a fairly leisurely descent down a gentle slope, even though I am used to rushing down steep inclines at a furious pace all year round. During my stay in the casualty hospital in Salzburg, one of the newest in Europe and, indeed, a showpiece, I had the opportunity of studying at close quarters, the excellent resources which our modern Western medicine has at its disposal for such cases. I was frequently asked what a traditional-style Asian healer would have done in a similar situation. I answered that, at all events, the local treatment would have been more difficult and also more painful, and under the best circumstances would probably have had approximately the same results. On the other hand however, additional methods would have been employed, such as the administration of suitable medicines, to speed up the knitting together of the bones 'from within'. A talented Tibetan doctor can reduce the time required by our methods for broken bones to heal to, let us say, two-thirds, using skilfully compounded medicines, which must also, however, be carefully adapted

[10] This has, indeed, now occurred to some extent with the introduction of Chinese medicine into Tibet. (Cf. *The Timely Rain, Travels in New Tibet* by Stuart and Roma Gelder, Hutchinson 1964.) (Tr.)

to the patient's whole constitution. The main constituents of such medicines are usually finely powdered transparent calcite and other minerals, combined with various admixtures necessary 'to dampen' the disadvantageous effect on the stomach often caused by such substances. Indeed, there are said to be special composite medications, which apparently speed up the healing process of broken bones even more. However, in view of possible unfavourable effects on various internal organs, their dispensation is subject to special precautions. Beyond this, the Tibetan healer would prepare a bonesetting pack, with medicinal plant extracts, to fix around the broken bones. These extracts – for example *stellaria media linn* (*cariophyllacaeae*), which grows in the heights of Western Tibet – would also contribute towards a quicker recovery.

This example demonstrates that practical co-operation with Tibetan physicians might even be possible in areas where our modern medicine has proved itself capable of great achievements.

*

The task is enormous but the goals are in sight. The first steps to bridge the gulf have been taken.

'Will a second Galen arise,' asks an old European medical textbook, 'who, like a great master builder of waterways, will encompass the divergent channels of the river of medicine and fuse them into a single powerful current?' This will not only depend on the good intentions, skill and spiritual level of particular individuals, but also on whether a humanity ensnared in suffering and sin is willing to enter upon the path towards new lines of thought and a new spiritual order. Thus the foundations of a new medicine may be created which in its essence will be neither specifically Eastern nor Western – an achievement heralding a new stage of development.

The Tibetan Art of Healing

Medicine can be totally different from what we are used to yet be effective, and Tibetan medicine is both – effective in many spheres and very, very different. Perhaps that is what makes it of wider interest at a time when many sense some lack of completeness in Western culture and seek out the global view. Here, in a broad perspective having general as well as technical significance, the author – who speaks Tibetan and studied with their practitioners – includes chapters on cancer, mental illness, and East-West research.